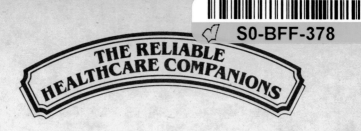

THE RELIABLE
HEALTHCARE COMPANIONS

This book and others in the series
have been prepared to give you a better
understanding of the disease. Armed with the
latest information on all aspects of
OSTEOPOROSIS, you will be in a better
position to prevent or minimize the problems
of this chronic illness.

Understanding
and
Managing
OSTEO-
POROSIS

EDITED BY
JOHN L. DECKER, M.D.
Director of the Clinical Center,
THE NATIONAL INSTITUTES OF HEALTH

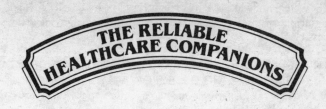

THE RELIABLE
HEALTHCARE COMPANIONS

Understanding
—and—
Managing

OSTEO-
POROSIS

EDITED BY
JOHN L. DECKER, M.D.
Director of the Clinical Center,
THE NATIONAL INSTITUTES OF HEALTH

AVON BOOKS 🔷 NEW YORK

The editor would like to thank Hugh Howard, John Gallagher, and Paul Cirincione, whose writing and research assistance helped make this series possible.

THE RELIABLE HEALTHCARE COMPANIONS: UNDERSTANDING AND MANAGING OSTEOPOROSIS is an original publication of Avon Books. This work has never before appeared in book form.

The medical and health procedures contained in this book are based on research recommendations of responsible medical sources. But because each person is unique, the author and publisher *urge the reader to check with his physician before implementing any of them.*

The author and publisher disclaim responsibility for any adverse effects or consequences resulting from the suggestions or the use of any of the preparations or procedures contained herein. No one should ever commence taking drugs or discontinue a prescribed drug regimen without first consulting a physician.

To our teachers and patients alike
this book is dedicated. So often,
the two are one and the same.

Table
of
Contents

A NOTE TO THE READER

Today, healthcare providers—doctors, nurses, and therapists—are beginning to accept the notion that the better informed the patient is, the more likely his or her condition is to improve. There has been, in fact, a clear movement in recent years to harness the patient's curiosity about his or her ailment and to put it to use in understanding its nature and treatment.

It was not always so. There was a time when the physician prescribed in Latin and was likely to respond to questions with knowing paternalism. ("Now, don't you worry about a thing.") Even today, doctors who are inclined to educate their patients find themselves so steeped in science and loaded with facts that to counsel the layperson is to walk a thin line between oversimplification and information overload.

On the other hand, we live in a world where the patient is offered unrealistic hopes of easy cures or instant pain relief by television advertising and media enthusiasm. We have come to believe that there is a harmless pill for every problem and that cures are the norm rather than the exception. While medical science has made incredible progress in understanding the structure and function of living things, there are still innumerable unanswered questions.

The fact is that, despite the pulsing excitement of research advances, we are today practicing what Dr. Lewis Thomas has called "a halfway technology." We are in a state of mildly confused uncertainty as to what is the preferable choice of action in many medical circumstances. It is this uncertainty, this contribution from many specialties, this clangor of divergent advice, to which THE RELIABLE HEALTHCARE COMPANIONS aim to bring some relief.

This book and the others in the series are meant to lead you in your quest for more knowledge, more help, and more support. Your illness may be confusing and its underlying causes obscure, but you'll want to understand what is happening to your body when you note changes in performance, appearance, or sensation. By using the resources identified here in conjunction with the guidance offered by your healthcare provider, you should develop a solid foundation for a counterattack upon your ailment. I wish you success.

John L. Decker, M.D.
Director, Warren Grant Magnuson Clinical Center
THE NATIONAL INSTITUTES OF HEALTH

PREFACE

Most people confronting a personal health problem like osteoporosis don't know where to begin.

This healthcare sourcebook differs from the other books on the market in that it is a catalogue of the kinds of help available for treating—and learning to live with—your osteoporosis. It will also give you the basics of what you need to know about the kind of osteoporosis you have.

Every patient with osteoporosis is a unique traveler through the medical landscape. There are no two patients who have the same manifestations, the same course, and the same qualitative and quantitative constellation of accompanying problems. But just as the same map can be given to and used by many travelers with many different destinations, so a single sourcebook of help can be relevant to a multitude of osteoporosis sufferers as they begin their patient education. You know best your unique problems and concerns; you do not have the same need for information, treatment, and support that your doctor's other patients do; your lifestyle will require unique adjustments that only you can identify and make.

But whatever your specific needs, in this book you will find:

- An authoritative yet accessible and comprehensive overview of the various types of osteoporosis, including answers to your questions regarding physical and emotional management, medications, and physical therapy;
- Key information about the role of specialists, community healthcare agencies, and patient support groups;
- Detailed advice on confronting and dealing with the day-to-day problems of osteoporosis through the use of nutritional therapies, exercise programs, and home healthcare equipment;
- An evaluation of the best available books and other publications about osteoporosis;
- A separate and detailed evaluation of audiovisual materials available for rent or purchase;
- Specific advice on how to get access to the above kinds of help (800 toll-free numbers, addresses, names).

Increasingly, the medical profession has come to acknowledge the value of patient education. Particularly with a chronic illness like osteoporosis, you as an educated patient can, with the cooperation of your doctor, use diet, medication, and exercise, as well as all the other resources now available to help control your ailment and make it more manageable.

Take advantage of the help in these pages, and of the innumerable sources of help out there; you don't have to fight osteoporosis alone.

Understanding and Managing
OSTEOPOROSIS

INTRODUCTION

Sometimes it seems as if diseases are like fads: one day an ailment you've never heard of before appears in the newspaper or comes up in conversation. Then you hear about it constantly.

AIDS is certainly one such disease and, to judge from press coverage, osteoporosis is another. Unlike AIDS, however, there's nothing new to osteoporosis, and, while it is not the terrible killer AIDS is, it often has crippling, painful effects.

Even worse, it affects as many as one in four American women over the age of forty-five, and about nine in ten over the age of seventy-five. One in three women now suffering from osteoporosis were affected by the age of fifty.

There are even more worrisome statistics. In 1986, 1.3 million fractures due to osteoporosis cost the nation between seven and ten billion dollars and caused forty thousand deaths.

What Is Osteoporosis?

As its name indicates, osteoporosis is a disease of the bones: it comes from the Greek *osteon* for "bone" and *porus* for "passage" or "pore." In the osteoporosis sufferer, the bones lose both their protein matrix and their calcium salt, making them less dense, more porous, and weaker.

Bones weakened by osteoporosis are more susceptible to fracture. In a patient with osteoporosis, daily occurrences that would have no effect on healthy bones can cause a broken bone. Sustaining a slight blow, falling, or simply lifting an object are all acts that wouldn't even bruise a normal person, but which can result in breakage in the osteoporosis sufferer.

To your doctor, osteoporosis actually refers to a variety of disorders. Each has much in common with the next, though their causes and treatments are often very different. In Chapter 1 we will talk about each of the varieties of osteoporosis.

1

How Do I Know if I Have Osteoporosis?

Except in advanced cases, answering this question is still a problem for your doctor. Bones will appear normal in an x-ray unless a third to a half of the calcium ordinarily deposited there has wasted away. There are some key symptoms, however, you should be alert for, and finding one or more of them is reason enough to go and see your doctor to establish whether you have osteoporosis. If you do, you and your doctor must develop a therapeutic program to limit further damage.

SYMPTOMS OF OSTEOPOROSIS

- Lower back pain.
- Loss of height: osteoporosis can cause you to grow shorter and your posture to become more stooped.
- Fractures of the hip, wrist, or vertebrae.
- Periodontal disease, especially pyorrhea, an inflammation of the gums.
- "Thin skin": if the skin on the back of your hand is loose and seems to lack pigments, you may have lost a body protein called collagen, which may also signal osteoporosis.

What Is Bone Loss?

The shape of the bone in an osteoporosis sufferer does not change, nor does the combination of ingredients that make up the bone. At its simplest, what occurs is a loss of bone.

Though they maintain the same outward shape, osteoporotic bones become less dense. An imbalance develops between the rate at which new bone is formed and the rate at which the calcium content of the bone is removed. While the normal body both builds and destroys bones by depositing or removing calcium salts, in the osteoporosis sufferer the withdrawals exceed deposits.

As the bones lose calcium, they become less dense. As the bones lose density, they lose strength. Weakened, osteoporotic bones become subject to fractures.

When Do I Call the Doctor?

If you suspect you have osteoporosis, the symptoms cited in these pages may help you. However, you must not rely on this or any book to provide you with a diagnosis. That is what your doctor is trained to do. If you think you have osteoporosis, make an appointment to see your physician. (If you do not have a doctor, see page 38 for advice about finding a suitable one.)

In fact, most osteoporosis is first diagnosed by doctors as a result of x-ray tests conducted to identify fractures or for some other purpose. Since osteoporosis may progress totally without symptoms and often is, consequently, unsuspected by the victim, an examination of the state of your bones and their degree of mineralization by x-ray may lead your physician to do further tests. (See Into the Laboratory, page 39.)

CHAPTER 1

The Disease

There are 206 bones of the human body. We tend to take our skeletons, as the framework of bones is called, for granted, paying them heed only when they break down. But the fact is that were it not for these rigid structures with their intermittent hinges, our bodies would be gelatinous lumps of flesh such as might be collected in a bushel basket or two. Our very shape and all our movements depend upon the skeleton.

Osteoporosis reduces the integrity of the skeleton by weakening its components. In order to understand osteoporosis, then, it is essential to understand bone: its ingredients, how they are combined, how the bone that results is maintained, and the other factors crucial to normal—and abnormal—bone.

The Normal Bone

Bones are composed of osseous tissue which, in turn, consists of three essential parts. First, there is the firm matrix made up of proteins and complicated sugars; second, there are minerals, principally hard, brittle crystals of calcium phosphate; third, there are the cells of bone, called osteocytes, osteoblasts, and osteoclasts.

One way to think of the ways these parts work together is to think of a clay sculpture. Usually the sculptor will make an armature of wire; then he will add clay to give that armature the shape he desires. The matrix and the minerals in your bones work together in a similar fashion.

Bones and sculptures, however, are unlike in that bones are alive and changing, in ways controlled by the bone cells mentioned above. First are the osteocytes, which maintain the osseous tissue and are probably involved in releasing calcium from bone

5

into the blood. The osteoblasts manufacture bone. They lay down the collagen (the principal protein in bone and in other connective tissues in the body) and the complex sugars to make the matrix. Then the calcium phosphate crystals assemble on that matrix. Osteoclasts produce powerful enzymes that are capable of digesting and destroying the matrix; the action of osteoclasts causes calcium crystals to be dislodged from the matrix and be dissolved for uses elsewhere or to be excreted. Thus, osteoclasts destroy bone. The osteoclast is able to remove all the bone deposited by 150 osteoblasts in a given period of time.

But don't think the osteoclasts are going to put you in a bushel basket. The fact is, fresh osseous tissue is deposited for every bit of bone removed and cut away in an unending process (the proper technical terms for the deposit and withdrawal of calcium are deposition and resorption). In children and adolescents, the deposition–resorption cycle is more active than in adults. Only about 3 percent of adult bone cells turns over in a typical year, while in youngsters the turnover is in the range of 100 percent per year (that is, all the existing bone is destroyed and replaced in that year).

One of the many miracles of our bodies is that this destruction and construction occur in balance. Though we don't understand how, our bodies keep the coming and going of calcium in a quite precise balance. When that balance is lost, osteoporosis may result.

Cortical and Trabecular Bone

We talked about the three constituent parts of bone tissue. Now we must introduce another complication: there are two kinds of bone tissue, both of which are made up of the same three bone parts. The two kinds of bone tissue are called cortical and trabecular bone.

When magnified many times, cortical bone looks (and is) solid. Trabecular bone, on the other hand, has the structure of a sponge or a honeycomb.

Different bones in the body are made up of different combinations of the two types of bone tissues. The shafts of the large leg and arm bones, for example, consist almost entirely of cortical bone, while the vertebral bones of the spinal column and the ends of the thigh bone (that is, the hip ball at the top and the spread out portion that meets the knee cartilage below) are made up largely of trabecular bone.

The patterns of the tiny struts in the sponge-like trabecular bone change in response to different loading or weight. If someone is fitted with an artificial limb, the use and directional forces of the good limb will change slightly. It has been observed that slowly, over a period of months, the trabecular bone will respond to the new forces and change alignment.

This is an important observation because it tells us the bone responds to physical forces upon it. The muscles of the body are all attached to bone, either directly or through cords of tissue called tendons. When the muscles contract, stress is put on the bone and the osseous tissue changes. This is true when we "bear weight," that is, stand up and put the weight of our body onto our feet and ankles. The stimulus and the response to it are critical to the maintenance of a healthy skeleton. We will discuss "weight-bearing" exercise and its potential benefits later in this book (page 110).

The deposition and resorption of bone is not a random process but occurs as a response to physical force. The remodeling of bone (that is, the coming and going, or deposition and resorption, of its mineral content) is at its most dramatic during the growth years of childhood and adolescence. The bones get heavier and wider: on the outer surfaces of the bones, cortical bone is added, while on the inner surfaces and spaces, the osteoblasts are at work making trabecular bone.

While the hollow inside the bones is free of bone, it isn't empty. The bone marrow found there is composed primarily of fat and hematopoietic tissue, the latter engaged in the production of the formed elements of blood, including red blood cells, white blood cells, and platelets. The bones are also supplied with blood vessels and nerves, the former bringing the "foodstuffs" and oxygen necessary for life. Even osteocytes, deep in a shell of self-maintained bone, are bathed by body fluids through which pass the chemicals without which they would die. They are relatively inactive cells, so they don't need as much nutrition as kidney cells, for example, but they need some. The fluids and cell water of bone, hard as it is, amount to almost half the weight of the bone.

Calcium:
The Key
Ingredient

In order to understand the bones of your body, you must also understand calcium.

Two to three pounds of your body weight is calcium, 99 percent of it in your bones and teeth. The other 1 percent is to be found in your soft tissues and circulating in the bloodstream.

The 1 percent of calcium that is not bone tissue performs a great variety of essential tasks throughout your body. Calcium is necessary for the normal functioning of the muscles (in particular, those of the heart) because it is crucial to the chemistry of muscular contraction and relaxation. Calcium is also involved in blood clotting, in activating certain enzymes, in stimulating insulin secretion, and in transmitting nerve impulses. Without calcium, we could not function.

Calcium is also a critical element in osteoporosis. Calcium makes the bones visible to x-rays; it gives the bones their hardness. It is its loss that weakens the bones in osteoporosis. So shouldn't treatment of osteoporosis simply be a matter of consuming more calcium to replace that which has been lost? In fact, the bodily processes involved are a good deal more complicated than that.

It's easy enough to think of eating calcium in the form of cheese or a pill, but one must be aware that only a part (that is, about half) of the calcium that is consumed is actually absorbed into the bloodstream. The other half is excreted.

Most of the calcium excreted goes out via the kidneys. In an hour-by-hour, short-term sense, it is kidney action which maintains the blood calcium within its normal levels. When a calcium-rich meal is eaten, calcium levels in the blood rise, and the kidneys respond by taking the calcium from the blood and putting it in the urine. If you choose to go on a crazy diet that contains no calcium—say, all fruit—the kidneys can reduce the urinary excretion of calcium to zero. Again, the precision of the correcting forces is a thing of beauty. It works because of a variety of factors, some of which we are coming to understand.

Factors in Maintenance of Blood Calcium

There are several key performers involved. Two are hormones: the thyroid gland provides one, calcitonin; the parathyroid glands provide another, parathormone. Another essential singer in the chorus is vitamin D, a nutrient found in a variety of dietary sources and formed in the skin upon exposure to sunlight. Let's look at them one at a time.

PARATHORMONE: When the level of calcium in your blood falls below normal levels, the four tiny parathyroid glands in the neck secrete parathormone into the blood. Parathormone causes your kidneys to retain calcium and your bones to release calcium into the bloodstream, helping to return calcium levels to normal.

VITAMIN D: Vitamin D is an unusual vitamin in that it more nearly resembles a hormone than other vitamins. It is derived from food sources (among them eggs, milk, and fish), but most of the body's supply is a product of the sun's interaction with an inactive form of the vitamin stored in the skin. After the vitamin is initially formed in the skin, it is activated in the liver and kidneys. When parathormone passes into the bloodstream, vitamin D responds to parathormone's particular tune: it relays the word to your intestines to absorb more calcium from the food you eat.

CALCITONIN: Calcitonin acts to stop the removal of calcium from your bones. When the level of calcium in your blood rises above normal levels, the thyroid gland secretes calcitonin, which alerts the bones to stop releasing calcium.

THE DATA ON VITAMIN D

FUNCTION: Vitamin D is essential to the tasks of absorbing calcium and phosphorus from the intestinal tract.

SYMPTOMS OF DEFICIENCY: The symptoms of a mild deficiency state are irritability and weakness; in the event of a severe deficiency, osteomalacia (softening of the bones) may occur. Symptoms include bone pain, especially in the legs, spine, and pelvis; anemia; and progressive weakness.

GOOD SOURCES: Butter, egg yolks, fish (in particular, those with fatty flesh, such as tuna, salmon, herring, and sardines), oysters, and liver.

RECOMMENDED DAILY INTAKE*:

Infants	400 international units
Children and adolescents 1 to 18 years of age	400 international units
Pregnant/lactating women	400 to 600 international units
Men and women 19 years of age and older	200 to 400 international units

*Source: Recommended Dietary Allowances, 9th ed., Food and Nutrition Board of the National Academy of Sciences/National Research Council, 1980.

Phosphorus: Calcium's Partner

Phosphorus and calcium are partners; they work together to form bones and teeth. Phosphorus helps your body use calcium effectively.

Like calcium, most of the phosphorus in the body is found in bone, roughly 85 percent. The rest is in muscles, skin, nerves, and other tissues.

Phosphorus has numerous uses in the body. It is essential for the use of carbohydrates, fats, and proteins. It is needed for the function of numerous enzymes. But in the context of osteoporosis, its most important role is in the development and maintenance of bone tissues.

While science understands a good deal about the coming and going of calcium from the bone, the regulation of phosphorus's movements is still largely a mystery. It is clear, however, that phosphorus is essential to the mineralization of bone.

The amount of phosphorus in our bodies varies with age. Its presence in the blood is high in childhood, then levels off. In men, the level of phosphorus in the blood gradually decreases into old age. In women, the pattern is different: the phosphorus level in the blood decreases through the twenties and thirties, but it rises again after age forty. Given the known correlation between an increase of phosphorus in the blood and of bone loss, it appears that the higher phosphorus levels in older women may be linked to the greater bone loss characteristic of those same women.

The fact is that too much phosphorus in the diet will inhibit calcium absorption. The two minerals will combine to form a compound called calcium phosphate. This compound cannot be absorbed and will be excreted, which effectively reduces the amount of calcium getting into the body.

For optimal calcium absorption, a dietary pattern that supplies roughly the same amounts of calcium and phosphorus is best. We will talk at length of how to go about achieving this balance in Chapter 4 (page 104).

In the following pages, we will talk at length about the absorption and utilization of calcium by your body. As the combination of interactions of calcitonin, vitamin D, phosphorus, and parathormone suggests, the process is extremely complex.

Bone Loss

Medicine is filled with complicated words. Thus, to a medical student, a bone that has lost density is showing "osteopenia." Bone loss is normal and inevitable after we reach age thirth-five, as the bones lose more calcium than is deposited. When calcium resorption (that is, removal of calcium from the bones) begins to exceed the rate at which calcium is deposited, there is a reversal of the trend characteristic of skeletal growth. It appears that bone loss is an unavoidable consequence of aging in both men and women. Osteoporosis is one kind of bone loss; osteomalacia is another.

Osteoporosis vs. Osteomalacia

While osteoporosis is a disease in which the body keeps an appropriate level of calcium in the blood at the expense of the bones, osteomalacia is a problem that results from insufficient absorption of calcium. People with osteomalacia (in children, the ailment is termed rickets) do not take in enough calcium from the intestines. Osteomalacia can be corrected by providing the body with an adequate supply of calcium and vitamin D. The mineral lost from the bones by the osteomalacia sufferer will be returned and the strength of the skeleton restored once the insufficiencies have been corrected.

Perhaps the key distinction between osteoporosis and osteomalacia is that in osteoporosis, the composition of the bone is normal—there is simply less of it. In osteomalacia, the amount of calcium stored in the bones is abnormally low.

Unfortunately, in osteoporosis the loss is irreversible in most cases. Osteoporosis is a more complex, chronic, and less understood problem.

"Condition" vs. "Disease"

Osteoporosis is more a condition than a "disease," and it is a term applied to bones which show decreased mass, that is, low density or less bone tissue. If one could take a small chunk of bone in the normal state and an identically sized piece of osteoporotic bone, there would be less bone tissue (collagen, matrix, crystals, cells, and all) in the latter piece, and it would weigh less than the normal one.

In treating patients, one finds that the bones of people with osteoporosis are less visible on x-rays. Because their bones are less dense, more of the x-rays pass through the bone and blacken the x-ray film. Instead of the normal, crisp white appearance, bones appear washed out, gray or mottled gray, with thin edges.

Osteoporosis has been termed a silent disease, since it may develop without outward signs or symptoms for many years before it is detected. Often the patient's first indication is a sudden bone fracture, one not precipitated by a major accident but in many cases by a simple strain or bump.

In some cases, fractures of the vertebrae, called "crush fractures" or "spinal compression fractures," are the first signs of osteoporosis. Surprisingly simple tasks like bending over to pick up an object—perhaps not even a heavy one—can lead to these vertebral fractures.

The result is usually a sudden pain in the back(though not always, as crush fractures can be painless). A gradual loss of height and a curvature of the upper spine, commonly referred to as a "widow's" or "dowager's hump," usually follow in the longer term. A loss in height of an inch and a half per decade after menopause is not uncommon as a result of these vertebral fractures.

Accompanying these changes will be persistent pain in the spine or the muscles that surround it. As portions of the spine collapse, more of the weight of the upper body must be borne by the muscles, and this added load may contribute to the pain. It is believed that the porous bone itself does not produce pain; rather, fractures of the bone, even tiny fractures of a few vertebrae that had previously gone unnoticed, cause the pain.

Am I at Risk?

How does the bone get into this deplorable condition? To answer this, we must go back to our idea of balance between bone formation and bone removal. To produce osteoporosis over the years, one needs to have reduced bone formation, increased bone destruction, or both. No one is quite sure which of these conditions exist, but the preponderance of medical opinion today is that there is a slight increase in the rate of bone destruction as we age. The osteoclasts, the cells that dissolve bone, appear to be too numerous and too vigorous in the patient with osteoporosis.

That osteoporosis is a potentially crippling disease is well known; the fact that its complications kill as many as 40,000 Americans each year is a terrible testament to its severity. At the very least, the osteoporosis sufferer is likely to find limits set on the kinds of physical activity he or she can perform. Pain and discomfort may also become constant companions.

There is good news, however. Much research activity has commenced in recent years into the causes and treatments of osteoporosis. This news should be especially encouraging to younger women who have the luxury of taking preventive measures in limiting their risks for the disease. So let us consider some of the issues germane to the development of osteoporosis.

Risk Factors

FEMALE SEX: Being female is an important risk factor, since women are much more likely to develop osteoporosis than men. There are a number of reasons, but a key one is that women start out with some 30 percent less bone mass than men.

OLDER AGE: The age factor is obviously important. In children and adolescents, the rate of calcium absorption is high, as up to 75 percent of dietary calcium is absorbed during periods of rapid skeletal growth. But by adulthood, only about 50 percent of the calcium from the diet is absorbed. At about age forty-five for women and age sixty for men, calcium absorption by the body decreases again due to changes in bowel function.

With a few notable exceptions, such as osteoporosis caused by the use of certain medications or by glandular abnormalities, osteoporosis is an ailment of older people. It also takes time for the effects of osteoporosis to become evident.

EARLY MENOPAUSE: Perhaps the single most important risk factor of all in women is the shortfall of estrogen that occurs following menopause, as we will see in the following pages. Women who experience menopause early—that is, before the age of forty-five—are more likely to get osteoporosis. This is particularly true if menopause was induced by the surgical removal of the ovaries or by other means; the loss produces a significant drop in estrogen output. One in four women who experience a natural menopause will develop osteoporosis, but of women who have their ovaries surgically removed, the chances double to nearly one in two. There are hormonal therapies, however, that can reduce this risk substantially (page 54).

On the other hand, it appears that women who have had children—and thereby experienced the high levels of estrogen during pregnancy that led to greater calcium absorption—may have a lesser risk of developing osteoporosis. The data on this is by no means definite as yet, so it would be an overstatement to suggest that pregnancy can prevent osteoporosis.

RACE: White men and women are more likely than black men and women to suffer from osteoporosis, as blacks have greater bone mass and seem to lose bone less rapidly. Some researchers go so far as to conclude that persons of British, Northern European, Chinese, or Japanese extraction are at greater risk than those of African, Hispanic, or Mediterranean descent.

LOW CALCIUM INTAKE: It is a simple equation: If you consume little calcium, there is little to be deposited in your bones. Studies also suggest that women with osteoporosis on average consume less calcium than healthy women of the same age. Low calcium consumption is common among the elderly in this country; older Americans are also more likely to be taking drugs that interfere with calcium absorption. To compound these factors, it is well known that the body's ability to absorb calcium declines after the age of forty, leading to more calcium passing directly through the body.

PHYSICAL INACTIVITY: Put simply, physical movement is necessary to the maintenance of the bones. Physical activity leads to increased bone mass (thus, athletes in general have greater bone mass than people who lead more sedentary lives). Patients who are bedridden or confined to wheelchairs for long periods are at greater risk for osteoporosis as, to a lesser extent, are those people who lead sedentary lives.

LOW BODY WEIGHT: The lesser bone mass characteristic of small body size seems to be another predisposition to the disease. In fact, it has been observed that obese women develop osteoporosis less often than slender women; one theory has it that the greater bulk of heavier women places greater stress on the bones, and they respond by developing more bone mass to meet the need.

Constant dieting (that is, the routine consumption of less than 1,500 calories a day) may lead to being underweight. It is also likely to result in a shortfall of essential calcium and other nutrients. A danger to the health of one's bones results.

FAMILY HISTORY: If others in your family have osteoporosis, you are at risk for developing it, too. In part, that is because your genes determine an upper limit for the growth of your bones. If the level of bone mass is not particularly high, you have less to lose and, therefore, your risk is greater.

ASSOCIATED DISEASES: A variety of other ailments are linked to osteoporosis. Among them are thyroid conditions and rheumatoid arthritis.

USE OF CERTAIN DRUGS: Numerous drugs, including corticosteroids, the anticoagulant heparin, and the anticonvulsant phenytoin (Dilantin), are known to contribute to the development of osteoporosis in some patients (pages 23-25). The diuretic furosemide (brand name: Lasix) also reduces body calcium.

Unlike some diseases for which cures have been found and about which the medical profession has a sense of having solved their mysteries, osteoporosis is new and not yet charted territory. Much time and many research dollars are, at present, being invested in its study, but many questions remain unanswered. Theories abound; proven scientific facts are not so numerous as we might like. The following are some of the areas being studied at present. These are thought to be risk factors for osteoporosis but are not yet proven to be.

SMOKING CIGARETTES: Although research findings have yet to prove that smoking is a direct cause of osteoporosis, it is true that a substantial percentage of women with osteoporosis smoke. Thus, smoking is thought to be a risk factor for osteoporosis in both men and women.

Smoking is also known to increase calcium loss from the bones. Another factor in the equation may be that women who smoke often reach menopause several years earlier than nonsmokers.

ALCOHOL ABUSE: Alcohol is a diuretic: as such, its consumption increases the flow of urine out of the body. In doing so, however, alcohol also causes increased excretion of calcium. In addition, alcohol also directly impairs the absorption of calcium. While it is not clear what level of alcohol intake is to be regarded as hazardous for calcium absorption, it does seem evident that alcoholics are at great risk, particularly since even young alcoholics have been found to develop osteoporosis. The lifestyle of many alcholics may also contribute to the development of osteoporosis, since a typical heavy drinker does not eat a balanced diet, does not get sufficient exercise, and may also suffer liver damage. In short, you should reduce your alcohol consumption to two drinks per day or less.

CAFFEINE CONSUMPTION: Like alcohol, caffeine is a diuretic and causes increased excretion of calcium. As a result, you should limit your consumption of foods, beverages, and medications containing caffeine as much as possible. No more than two cups of coffee or tea should be drunk daily.

USE OF ANTACIDS: Research suggests that aluminum- and magnesium-based antacids increase excretion of calcium. This occurs because these antacids lower blood phosphorous levels, causing phosphorous to be liberated from the bones to maintain blood levels. Because phosphorus is removed from the bones along with calcium, bone calcium is reduced.

You should avoid taking aluminum-based antacids in particular for a prolonged period; switching to a calcium-based antacid might be a suitable solution.

ARE YOU AT RISK FOR OSTEOPORSOSIS?

There is no proven formula for anticipating who will and who will not develop brittle bones, but the following are known risk factors:

- Female sex: Women are seven times as likely to be affected as men.
- Older age: In general, osteoporosis is an ailment apparent in women over the age of fifty and men over the age of seventy.
- Early menopause (natural or surgical): Menopause means the cessation of estrogen secretion, a key ingredient in the calcium absorption equation.
- Race: White men and women are more likely to suffer from osteoporosis than black men and women.
- Low calcium intake (less than 450 mg daily): The less calcium there is in your diet, the less there is to absorb.
- Sedentary lifestyle: Exercise is critical in building and maintaining bone tissues; in particular, if you are largely immobile, your risk of osteoporosis is great.
- Slight build: The less bone mass you have to start with, the more severe the effects of decreased bone density will be.
- Family history: Many persons with osteoporosis come from families in which there have been other members with the disease.
- Drug use: Long-term use of corticosteroids, the anticonvulsant phenytoin (Dilantin), the anticoagulant heparin, and antacids that contain aluminum have been shown to lead to osteoporosis.
- Cigarette smoking: Smokers tend to reach menopause earlier, and tobacco may have an effect on the body's ability to use vitamin D, a crucial element in the absorption of calcium.
- Excessive alcohol consumption: Alcohol is a diuretic, so consuming it means that you will excrete calcium you might otherwise absorb.

Menopause

Recent studies indicate that the decrease in estrogen levels in women due to menopause may be, along with a low level of calcium consumption, one of the most critical factors in the development of osteoporosis.

Menopause, also known as "change of life" or "climacteric," is, at its simplest, the time of life marked by the permanent cessation of menstruation. It occurs to one in four American women by about the age of forty-five; by age fifty-five, 95 percent will have experienced menopause.

Perhaps the most common symptom of menopause is hot flashes or flushes. A hot flush is a feeling of heat that comes on suddenly and spreads over all or a portion of the body. Blushing or sweating may accompany the sensation. Flushes often occur at night and may disrupt sleep.

Other symptoms of menopause are feelings of physical weakness, vaginal dryness, and, in some cases, mental depression. Menstruation itself may cease quite suddenly, flow may decrease over a period of months, or the cycle may increase in length until flow ceases entirely. Menopause may also be induced by the surgical removal of the ovaries.

The key factor in the menstrual equation is the hormone estrogen. Like other hormones, estrogen acts as a chemical messenger that, after traveling through the bloodstream to another part of the body, stimulates increases in activity. Secreted by the ovaries, estrogen controls the development and maintenance of female sexual characteristics.

Menstruation occurs because estrogen stimulates cyclic changes in the lining of the vagina and uterus. When the ovaries begin producing estrogen at puberty, menstruation begins. Loss of ovarian estrogen production, signaled by the cessation of menstruation, is the cause of menopause.

Estrogen has a wide variety of other effects on the body. Though it is not well understood, it is thought that one such function is to control—or at least strongly influence—the formation of the bones by speeding or slowing bone loss. Estrogen may also affect the bowel's ability to absorb calcium from the diet. The bones do not interact directly with estrogen, but estrogen does play an important role in controlling levels of parathormone, vitamin D, and calcitonin, all of which have essential calcium-related functions (page 9).

These apparent influences on the presence of calcium in the body are consistent with the changing needs of a woman of child-bearing years. When carrying a child, the skeleton needs to be extra strong; as the fetus develops and, after birth, during breast feeding, additional calcium is also required. To meet these needs, a reserve of calcium is maintained, thanks to the effects of estrogen.

After a woman reaches menopause, her need for extra calcium to meet the special requirements of childbearing and nursing cease. Because this reserve of calcium is no longer necessary—and since the high levels of estrogen that led to its accumulation decrease—her bones will contribute a large portion of the calcium required to maintain normal body functions.

These factors and others discussed in the following pages result in bones becoming progressively more porous and brittle. In people who develop osteoporosis, this process proceeds at a faster than normal rate.

The Varieties of Osteoporosis

The varieties of osteoporosis all share one key characteristic: a net loss of bone resulting in osteopenia. The mechanism of this withering of bone differs from one variety to the next.

In medicine, the talk is often of "etiology"; to the layperson, the word more often used is "cause" (or "causes"). Beginning with differences in cause, distinctions can be drawn regarding the varieties of osteoporosis.

Primary Osteoporosis

The vast majority of osteoporosis patients suffer from primary osteoporosis, a broad category that includes two, more narrow-ly defined subclassifications of osteoporosis.

The first occurs primarily in women aged fifty-five to seventy-five and is called "postmenopausal osteoporosis." It is thought to be a result of changes at menopause and is, therefore, likely to be treated with hormone therapies. The second, termed "senile osteoporosis," is believed to be, in part, a product of a shortfall of dietary calcium; it occurs primarily in men and women aged seventy to eight-five.

Given that these two varieties closely resemble each other and have many of the same causes, our discussion often will address them as one form termed primary osteoporosis. However, when distinguishing between the two is important, we will refer to the relevant variety specifically as postmenopausal or senile osteoporosis.

The principal consequence of both varieties of primary osteoporosis is the severe loss of bone mass. Given that, in general, bone loss begins earlier in women and since women have less bone mass to start with, it follows naturally that primary osteoporosis is more likely to occur—and to occur earlier—in women than in men.

On the other hand, the cause of the bone loss is unknown. There are a number of plausible theories, but none can yet be said to have been proven. The cessation of estrogen production by the ovaries at menopause seems the most obvious cause, but it seems an incomplete explanation since women who have their ovaries removed surgically do not all develop osteoporosis (though they do seem to be at roughly twice the risk of doing so than are women who undergo a natural menopause).

A shortfall of calcium in the body, caused by inadequate dietary intake or problems with absorption, may cause senile osteoporosis and contribute to postmenopausal osteoporosis. Here again, however, it seems that this is more likely to be but a contributory cause, given that many people with chronic low intakes of calcium or with absorption problems do not develop the disease.

Thus, the best guess medicine has to offer today is that a combination of factors is most likely responsible for primary osteoporosis. They are fourfold: one, insufficient bone mass generation during adolescence; two, inadequate calcium consumption; three, the decreasing ability of the bowels to absorb calcium as we age; and four, hormonal changes, in particular those occurring after menopause. Describing a recent conference on the subject at the National Institutes of Health, a *New York Times* headline writer summed it up nicely: "Dozens of Factors Critical in Bone Loss Among Elderly."

Endocrine Osteoporosis

Our glands constitute our endocrine system. The glands secrete hormones directly into the bloodstream or lymph system and then are circulated to other parts of the body. The hormones act as messengers, instructing other tissues to perform various functions.

People with endocrine disorders of great rarity, such as acromegaly or Cushing's syndrome, or somewhat more common problems such as hyperthyroidism or hyperparathyroidism, all are at risk of accelerated osteoporosis.

Acromegaly: Also referred to as acromegalia, this chronic disease of middle-aged adults is characterized by the gradual growth of the hands, feet, jaw, and skull bones. It results from an overactivity of the pituitary gland. Often the most noticeable change in a patient with acromegaly is the exaggerated growth of the forehead and jawbones, producing enlarged and coarsened facial features and widely separated teeth. While osteoporosis occasionally develops in patients with acromegaly, it is relatively rare.

Cushing's Syndrome: On the other hand, those who suffer from Cushing's syndrome commonly suffer from osteoporosis. Cushing's syndrome is caused by an overproduction of hormones by the adrenal glands or by prolonged use of corticosteroid drugs. (See Corticosteroids, page 24.)

Symptoms include fatigue, cessation of menstruation, impotence, edema (water retention), excess hair growth, and osteoporosis. Often the bone loss is most noticeable in the spine and pelvis.

HYPERTHYROIDISM: Hyperthyroidism is commonly referred to as an overactive thyroid. The excessive production of hormones by the thyroid gland increases the body's normal pace (that is, its "basal metabolic rate") and increases the appetite. The result, however, is often weight loss, nervousness, sweating, increased heart rate, and goiter, an enlargement of the thyroid gland that appears as a swelling in the neck.

Often hyperthyroidism also results in demineralization of the bones, which can lead to fractures. Readily available drug and surgical treatments are effective in treating both the hyperthyroidism and its side effect, osteoporosis.

HYPERPARATHYROIDISM: This condition is due to overactivity of the parathyroid glands, four small assemblages of tissue embedded in the thyroid gland at the base of the throat. Excessive hormone may be secreted due to a tumor or for unknown reasons. The results, however, are a notable increase in the amount of calcium in the blood and urine, and a lessened amount of phosphorus. The usual symptoms of hyperparathyroidism are muscle weakness, easy fatigue, constipation, and other digestive discomforts. Treatment is by radiation or surgical therapy of the gland and its affected tissue.

Drugs That Can Cause Osteoporosis

PHENYTOIN: The anticonvulsant medication phenytoin (better known by its brand name, Dilantin) interferes with the body's ability to metabolize vitamin D, a key player in the absorption of calcium (see page 9). The long-term use of Dilantin has been known to produce not only osteomalacia but problems that closely resemble osteoporosis.

HEPARIN: Heparin is an anticoagulant drug (commonly referred to as a blood thinner). It is given to patients with arteriosclerosis, or "hardening of the arteries," because their blood tends to clot more easily than normal, a condition that can result in the blockage of vessels. If such clotting occurs in the brain or heart, a stroke or heart attack can occur.

When injected in large amounts for six months or more, heparin may cause osteoporosis. If osteoporosis develops, the drug should be withdrawn and another anticoagulant substituted. If you are taking heparin and suspect osteoporosis, inform your physician. In most cases, the bones will recover lost calcium over time after the drug is discontinued.

CORTICOSTEROIDS: Use of corticosteroids can also result in osteoporosis. They are synthetic hormones that closely resemble the hormones secreted by the adrenal glands, and they have very potent anti-inflammatory effects. There are a great many brand names under which corticosteroid drugs are sold, but some of the generics are hydrocortisone, dexamethasone, methylprednisolone, prednisolone, and prednisone.

Regarded as miracle drugs when they were first introduced, they still can be called upon to produce miraculous results in treating a variety of illnesses—including arthritis, skin ailments, allergies, adrenal gland deficiencies, and some acute catastrophes—but we now know that their long-term use produces a number of hazardous side effects. Calcium loss is one of them. (See also Cushing's syndrome, page 22).

Corticosteroids, also referred to as glucocorticoids or simply just steroids (a commonly used, though slightly inaccurate nickname), decrease the absorption of calcium, in part because they interfere with the body's ability to produce vitamin D. They also increase resorption of calcium from the bones.

The degree of calcium loss is most closely tied to the length of time over which the drug is used rather than to the dosage. Short-term use of corticosteroids may produce osteomalacia; long-term use may result in osteoporosis.

If you are taking corticosteroid drugs and develop osteoporosis, your physician is likely to reduce the dosage to less than 10 milligrams a day and may instruct you to take the medication on alternate days. Do not, however, adjust the dosage yourself, because when you take these hormones orally over a long period, they replace the function of your own adrenal and pituitary glands. As a result, those glands will tend to atrophy or "go to sleep."

A weakened, collapsed state can result from abruptly stopping corticosteroid medications. Though the safety margin is great, they should only be reduced or stopped as directed by your doctor.

OTHER DRUGS: The following drugs are not likely to be the principal cause of anyone's osteoporosis. However, because they have an impact upon your body's ability to use calcium, you should use them with caution if you have osteoporosis or are at risk for the disease.

Some drugs of the class known as diuretics interfere with the absorption of dietary calcium so that more of the mineral is excreted. As a result, your body is likely to liberate calcium from the bones to maintain normal blood calcium levels. Furosemide (brand name: Lasix) can contribute significantly over time to calcium loss. If you take furosemide, discuss with your doctor the effect it has on your bones. It may make sense to change your medication to one of the thiazide diuretics which do not lead to calcium loss.

Antacids containing aluminum or magnesium can also lead to excretion of valuable calcium. Try switching to one that contains calcium; it may actually help, as the calcium in the antacid will supplement your dietary sources. (See discussion of calcium supplementation, page 60).

Miscellaneous Causes of Osteoporosis

Osteoporosis can result from causes other than normal aging, endocrine disorders, and the use of certain drugs. Such causes include immobilization, cancer, and various other disorders.

IMMOBILIZATION: Often called "disuse osteoporosis," this variety of osteoporosis results from prolonged immobilization of a limb following trauma: a broken arm or leg, its movements frozen in a cast for months, may lose calcium. Disuse osteoporosis generally affects only those bones that have been immobilized, whether due to a cast or some type of paralysis.

The loss of bone tissue results from a massive increase in the removal of calcium from the bones. The calcium is not replaced as it ordinarily would be because there is no stress put on the bone by normal use—once again, the importance of weight-bearing exercise is pointed out. In addition to the risk of osteoporosis caused by this wholesale withdrawal of calcium from the bones, there is also a danger of too much calcium in the blood or elsewhere in the body. To prevent calcium from accumulating in the kidneys, patients who are immobilized for prolonged periods are often required to increase their intake of fluids and are provided extensive physical therapy.

GENETIC CAUSES: Osteogenesis imperfecta is an inherited disease in which the bones develop imperfectly. In some cases, fractures are present even at birth. Recurrent fractures are the rule in patients with osteogenesis imperfecta.

Homocystinuria, an inherited disease characterized by mental retardation, has a variety of physical manifestations, among them osteoporosis. Patients with homocystinuria often experience fractures, as their bones lack calcium due to the absence of an enzyme required for the formation of collagen, the key protein of bone.

Other inherited ailments characterized by problems of connective tissues and, with them, collagen and bone, include Marfan syndrome, Ehlers-Danlos syndrome, Menkes syndrome, and Riley-Day syndrome. All are relatively rare but are in some cases accompanied by osteoporosis.

JUVENILE OSTEOPOROSIS: Also called "idiopathic" osteoporosis (because its cause is unknown), juvenile osteoporosis is a rare disorder. It occurs in children before puberty, usually between the ages of eight and fourteen. The characteristic symptom is bone pain, though fractures may also occur. Usually the disorder disappears as the child ages, and most children recover entirely within five years. Treatment is usually limited to avoiding excessive weight gain and minimizing immobilization.

OTHER CAUSES: Osteoporosis also occurs in some patients suffering from rheumatoid arthritis, certain obstructive lung diseases, Type I insulin-dependent diabetes, and chronic liver disease. To judge by the frequency with which the bone wasting occurs in conjunction with these ailments, it appears that pure chance is not an adequate explanation. Yet scientists have yet to explain why the pairings occur.

Other diseases that can share symptoms of osteoporosis include osteomalacia (page 12) and certain forms of cancer, such as cancer that has spread to the bones. Your doctor will conduct various laboratory tests to be sure those disorders are not present.

Malabsorption of calcium can also occur as a result of impaired function of the small intestine, liver, or pancreas. Again, relatively simple laboratory tests can be conducted to exclude this cause. If a high level of calcium is found in the urine, a malabsorption problem is probably not present, since too much calcium in the urine may be seen in primary osteoporosis.

Complications

By itself, the loss of bone mass wouldn't be of particular significance; the problems occur because the loss of mass also means an accompanying loss of bone strength. Bone fractures and deformities can be the painful and debilitating result.

Not all broken bones in the elderly are the direct result of osteoporosis. Reduced vision, episodes of dizziness, and fainting are common in older persons and can lead to falls that might not produce fractures in younger bones. But as we age, our bones grow more brittle, making them more subject to fracture upon trauma so mild that it would not damage a normal individual.

We talked earlier of the two kinds of bone tissue, the very hard cortical bone and the softer, honeycombed trabecular bone. It is the latter that is most likely to be affected by osteoporosis. Its honeycombed configuration gives the trabecular bone much greater surface area from which calcium can be withdrawn. While the more dense cortical bone tends to demineralize less than the trabecular bone, over time it, too, thins and weakens.

Bone Fractures

The susceptibility of the trabecular bone to calcium loss results in greater weakness in those bones with higher percentages of trabecular bone tissue. The vertebrae and the ends of the long bones of the leg and arm are thus most likely to be weakened. The result is that the areas of the body most often subject to fracture in the osteoporosis sufferer are the wrist, spine, and hip.

Any bone can be affected, but as these sites are the most likely to be affected, we will discuss each of them in detail.

WRIST FRACTURES: The "radius" or wrist bone is often fractured in the osteoporosis patient in what is called a "Colles fracture." The most common cause is a fall: upon instinctively reaching out to break one's fall, the hand and wrist absorb the shock. If the wrist bones are weakened by osteoporosis, a fracture often results.

The shorter but thicker of the two bones in the lower arm, the radius, is composed of about 25 percent trabecular bone at its lower end. With the loss of both the trabecular and the cortical bone through osteoporosis, the radius is weakened, making it susceptible to fractures. As is often the case with bone problems like this one, wrist breaks are much more common among older women than older men: women over age fifty are almost ten times as likely to break a wrist than men of the same age.

Usually, the prognosis for total recovery after a broken wrist is very good. The bones tend to heal relatively easily, and long-term disability is not common. However, such a fracture can be an early indication of bone loss. If you have experienced a broken wrist and are unsure of the status of your bones, it would be wise to consult with your physician regarding preventive treatments for osteoporosis.

VERTEBRAL FRACTURES: The human backbone consists of thirty-three vertebrae. Each vertebra is a shaped block of bone that fits into discs above and below; stacked together, they form the spine. A complex of ligaments, cartilage, and muscle hold the vertebrae in position.

The vertebrae are 90 percent trabecular bone and thus are especially susceptible to loss of bone mass. In fact, in osteoporosis patients, vertebral fractures may be produced by lifting a heavy object or by less strenuous events: even riding in a car on a bumpy road has been reported to cause vertebral fractures. In many cases, the breaks even occur spontaneously, with no apparent event having precipitated them.

In more than half of those who suffer them, fractures of the vertebrae go unnoticed when they occur. The area of the fracture is, however, tender to the touch and may, over time, produce backache. Most often, the fractures and the back pains are in the lower back. While the pains do not usually extend into other areas, they are often constant and worsened by bending and lifting. Many patients find that the pain can be relieved only by remaining motionless in bed, lying on one's side with knees and hips flexed. Sitting or standing for long periods often intensifies the pain.

Though in some cases a dull, constant "nagging" pain may remain indefinitely, more often the pain will decrease and disappear over a period of weeks. Muscle weakness and fatigue are likely to be present during that time.

The pain will recur if another vertebral compression fracture occurs. The eventual result of a series of such crush fractures in the osteoporosis patient is a loss of body height: literally, the sufferer will become shorter in stature and often assume a bent-over or "humpback" posture. Five vertebrae that have had crush fractures may take up the space previously filled by only three.

The "dowager's" or "widow's" hump is not the inevitable result of vertebral fractures. The progression of the disease varies. The pain may be constant and radiate to the abdomen or thighs, or there may be no pain at all. Generally, though, one vertebral fracture will be followed by others, usually within several years. In some cases, the increasingly bent-over posture will also produce a downward tilt to the rib cage, which in turn may result in a protruding abdomen. This is the result of the rib cage displacing internal organs, causing them to stick out. This is likely to be a painful process.

The older you get, the more likely you are to have osteoporosis in the spine. Recent studies suggest that the spines of almost a third of women between the ages of forty-five and fifty-five are affected; that in those age fifty-five to sixty-five, the chances of spinal involvement are nearly two out of three; and that in those age sixty-five and older, the chances are almost 80 percent.

HIP FRACTURES: Broken hips are common among the elderly: nearly 200,000 Americans sustain broken hips each year, an untold number of them as a result of osteoporosis. In fact, hip fractures are the most serious consequence of the bone loss that occurs in osteoporosis.

If you have sustained wrist or vertebral fractures, it appears that you are at higher risk for the more severe hip fracture. In fact, your doctor may even recommend an occupational therapy evaluation of your home and lifestyle to try and reduce the hazards that could cause you to sustain a hip fracture. (See discussion of the occupational therapist's role, page 84.)

A fall can cause the upper portion of the thigh bone to break, but in the osteoporosis patient, a less violent occurrence—even a shifting of weight—can cause a break. In some cases, it appears that a fall caused the break, when in fact the fracture occurred first and led to the fall.

The upper portion of the thigh bone contains a larger proportion of trabecular bone than the lower portion. As a result, patients with osteoporosis are most likely to experience substantial loss of bone tissue in the so-called head and neck of the thigh bone, the portions near the hip joint. The cortical bone on the outside thins and weakens, and the honeycombed trabecular bone within also becomes less dense. Hip fractures, as a consequence, become much more likely. To make matters worse, hip fractures frequently strike twice, affecting one and then the other hip.

Hip fractures do not heal as routinely as wrist breaks do; unlike crush fractures of the spine, they may limit mobility for more than a few days. In fact, only about half of the women who suffer hip fractures regain full, normal function. One in six dies shortly after her injury, and almost one in three within a year.

The usual treatment for a hip fracture is surgical repair of the hip joint, using screws or metal pins. In some cases, a hip replacement is required. (See Surgery, page 65.) The duration of the hospital stay is likely to be three to six weeks, though the period of recovery can extend for months, often necessitating confinement in a nursing home or other situations where nursing care is available. This is also an important time to gain help from occupational and physical therapists (see page 84). Among the major missions is the restoration of walking ability.

The fractures themselves do not cause death. Rather, complications stemming from the extended confinement are the usual cause. Pneumonia, blood clots, and fat embolisms (bone marrow fat that becomes trapped in the lungs) are the killers.

Blood clots occur because the hip operation and the consequent swelling of tissue about the hip partially obstructs the flow of blood in the large leg veins. A condition called phlebothrombosis can result: blood clots form along the inside of vessels, slowing the flow of blood and in some cases roughening the vessel walls. When least expected, or perhaps on the first effort to walk, a large piece of clot will be knocked loose, dragged by the blood to the heart, and pumped by the heart into the blood vessels of the lung. The moving clot is called an embolus, and the process is referred to as embolization. The result is the death of lung tissue, an event called a pulmonary infarction, which can be fatal within minutes.

Two measures are taken to prevent blood clots: early efforts to get the patient walking and the administration of anticoagulant drugs. The latter tends to block clot formation in the blood vessels. The former is practiced so early as to seem cruel, but the purpose is sound.

The Future

If osteoporosis can be regarded as a riddle, then we are still looking for the clues that will enable us to unscramble it. We don't quite understand why it occurs in one patient but not the next—even though the profiles of the two seem identical. We aren't really sure of precisely how to use each of the treatments at our disposal: one treatment may work for some patients but do nothing for others. At this moment, at least, osteoporosis presents us with a multitude of mystifying aspects.

On the other hand, in the last decade we have seen an enormous increase in our understanding of the ailment. In part, changing demographics and increasing population age have forced the collective hand of the medical profession: tens of millions of Americans have osteoporosis, and those of us who practice medicine see them every day. We are conducting many studies of the factors that cause or influence the development of osteoporosis; week after week medical journals tell us what researchers are learning about calcium supplements and the value of exercise and of experimental drugs and treatments.

One result of the past few years of intensive study of osteoporosis is an increasing awareness of what we don't know: we can direct our energies more effectively proceeding into areas where we know work is needed. The following are several of those major concerns.

DIAGNOSTIC TECHNIQUES: One area where advances are much needed is in screening patients for osteoporosis: too many sufferers come to us with fractures, entirely unaware that osteoporosis has been eroding their skeletons for years.

We need methods for determining earlier that bone loss is occurring. In Chapter 2 (page 39), we will talk about state-of-the art laboratory tests for determining bone mass. Testing methods are improving, but at present we don't have anything like a foolproof testing apparatus.

MEDICATIONS: At the moment, there is no miracle potion that, upon consumption, will make weakened bones strong again.

On the other hand, research is continuing at a rapid rate on a number of fronts. Synthetic versions of estrogen hormones, vitamin D, and calcitonin are being used to treat osteoporosis, as are the mineral boron and other substances. Fluoride, the same substance used to prevent tooth decay, is also being used in experiments on patients with osteoporosis. There are successes being reported and new drugs on the horizon—along with risks and failures.

PREVENTION: One key responsibility that the medical profession has is to try and help people avoid disease. Sometimes it's a matter of telling the sun-sensitive patient not to bake on the beach. We tell people to quit smoking or to cut down on their alcohol consumption or to lose weight. None of these advisories comes with any guarantees, of course, but an ever-growing body of research argues for their value in preventing skin cancers and emphysema and liver and heart disease and other problems.

Osteoporosis, we are finding, is no different. Today we can help many patients control their osteoporosis; tomorrow, we hope to be able to help them more, even cure them. But the most important goal before us is to help protect millions of men and women from developing the disease.

We are learning more about how to do it. In Chapter 2, we will discuss at length some techniques both of prevention and treatment. Although osteoporosis is not solely a matter of lifestyle—some people, regardless of how little milk they drink, will never experience a vertebral fracture—the chances of avoiding its pains and disabilities can be substantially reduced by following some of the strategies outlined in the chapter that follows. Read and learn about these strategies—then put them to use.

CHAPTER 2

Care and Treatment

The subject of this chapter is what is known today about caring for the osteoporosis patient and treating his or her ailment. In Chapter 1, a number of treatments were referred to; it is in this chapter that we will describe them in detail. Further, because there is a growing body of scientific evidence that suggests osteoporosis can be prevented or, at least, its worst effects can be limited, we will discuss how the premenopausal woman can try to make up for the bone loss of later years.

Osteoporosis is a chronic condition: the sufferer has to live with osteoporosis for life. While many patients can live quite normal lives, a comprehensive program of exercise, bone protection, and medication or food supplements is in order for virtually all osteoporosis patients. In some cases, surgery and physical therapy are also required.

The facts are that many women get osteoporosis and that the older you are, especially if you have passed through menopause, the more likely you are to suffer the irreversible bone loss of osteoporosis. Yet osteoporosis is not simply a matter of age. It occurs in relatively young people (especially alcoholics), and it does not happen to everybody. It appears that osteoporosis is, to no small degree, a result of the body's natural changes.

We talked at length in the previous chapter about the changes wrought in women during menopause, specifically on their ability to absorb and use calcium. That is perhaps the signal event in the osteoporosis story, but there are a number of other age-related factors as well.

As we age, we tend to eat less calcium-rich food. Science as yet cannot explain why, but our dietary habits change. The senses of smell and taste deteriorate. Our stomachs produce less hydrochloric acid, which affects our digestion. This, along with other changes in the digestive tract, may interfere with our ability to absorb calcium. In many people, dental problems make chewing more difficult, and frequently we lose our taste for milk and dairy products.

The amount of vitamin D we absorb also decreases as we age. In addition, many older people find themselves housebound or otherwise limit their exposure to the sun; as a result, less of this key vitamin is formed in the skin. A shortfall of vitamin D, as we discussed in the previous chapter (page 9), will lead to a decrease in calcium absorption.

As we age, we tend to become less active, which leads to less calcium deposition in the bones. Our basal metabolic rate—that is, the rate at which the body uses energy while at rest—decreases as we reach middle age and older. We respond by eating less in order to maintain our weight, often by eliminating foods that are rich in calories, like calcium-rich dairy products.

The upshot of these and other factors is that millions of Americans do not consume enough calcium. According to a report in the *Journal of the American Dietetic Association,* the daily intake of older men on average is less than 800 milligrams a day (the Recommended Dietary Allowance is 1,000 milligrams). Even more significantly, this ten-state study revealed that older women, who should be consuming 1,500 milligrams a day, consumed even less calcium than the men. Other studies have found that vitamin D consumption is similarly low.

There is no one therapeutic program that is right for all osteoporosis patients, nor is there likely to be complete agreement among researchers about the right way to treat any individual case. However, determining the exact course of care and treatment for you should be the result of an ongoing collaborative effort between you and your doctor. The first key step in the process, then, for the osteoporosis patient is to find the right professional guidance; but before we discuss finding a doctor, let's talk about what can be done even earlier to prevent bone loss.

Prevention

Osteoporosis research is proceeding at a rapid rate. Both the medical profession and the lay public have become acutely aware in recent years of how serious and widespread a health problem the disease is. Much energy is being invested in trying to understand its mysteries, but innumerable questions remain unanswered.

When it comes to prevention, it may take many, many years before we can be confident in asserting what behavioral measures help prevent the occurrence of osteoporosis. Although we lack solid proof, many researchers are confident that certain steps can be taken, especially by young and middle-aged women, to avoid the worst complications of the disease in later life.

Peak Bone Mass

The best current wisdom has it that the chances of avoiding osteoporosis are best when one has achieved a high peak bone mass. "Peak bone mass" is the point at which one's bones have accumulated their maximum mass and, consequently, their maximum strength. Since it usually occurs at about thirty-five years of age, by assuring that that peak bone mass is high, one may well be acting to reduce the chances of osteoporosis in later years. This is likely to be true of men as well as women.

CONSUME SUFFICIENT CALCIUM: One way to achieve maximum bone mass is to consume adequate calcium in your diet. A variety of evidence for this exists. One study conducted in Yugoslavia found that bone density was high among young people who lived in a district where a relatively high amount of calcium was consumed, while young residents of another district with lower calcium consumption had lower bone mass.

If you cannot consume the Recommended Dietary Allowance of calcium in your diet, take calcium supplements. (See page 61 for discussion of whether to supplement or not, and page 100 for discussion of dietary sources of calcium.)

ESTROGEN REPLACEMENT THERAPY: For nearly thirty-five years, estrogens have been used to treat osteoporosis. While researchers advocate their use only under certain circumstances, there is substantial evidence that they can prevent fractures and height loss.

During menopause, the ovaries cease to produce estrogen. As we discussed in Chapter 1, this has a substantial impact on the body's ability to absorb and store calcium. In order to limit the amount of calcium that is lost as the estrogen supply slows and eventually stops, your doctor may well prescribe estrogen replacement therapy (ERT) if you are at high risk for developing osteoporosis.

We will discuss at length later in this chapter the use of estrogen supplements by women during menopause as both a preventive for osteoporosis and a treatment. (See Medication, page 46.)

EXERCISE PROGRAMS: It is also important to get ample weight-bearing exercise. There seems to be an emerging consensus that three to four hours per week of weight-bearing exercise may be crucial not only to treating osteoporosis but to preventing it. To that end, in Chapter 4 we will discuss at length appropriate kinds of exercise for the young person concerned with avoiding bone loss in the coming years as well as exercise for the older individual who has already sustained such losses. (See Exercise Programs, page 110.)

It is also advisable to avoid behavioral risk factors like smoking and alcohol abuse. (See page 17 for explanations of these and other risk factors.) Together, these strategies may help prevent osteoporosis.

Selecting a Doctor

Living with a serious disease without a doctor is like driving a car without knowing how. It can be done, of course, but the risks are great.

Each case of osteoporosis is different from the next. A doctor is crucial in determining the nature of your case as well as in devising a suitable treatment program.

As the rest of this chapter points out, there are a multitude of treatments available. Some are as simple as eating more calcium-rich foods and involve measures that let you live as normally as possible. Others involve surgery and unusual medications. But negotiating the tricky terrain of the medical landscape requires a tour guide. Enter your family physician.

The best place to start dealing with your osteoporosis is with a doctor who knows you. If you think you have osteoporosis, make an appointment to see your family physician.

In Chapter 3 we will discuss the specialists and when they are to be consulted, but in many cases of osteoporosis, the expenditure of time and money to visit specialists is not required. Instead, it is your family doctor who can provide you with the guidance and treatment you need.

If you have no regular physician, inquire of friends or relatives about who they see when they have a medical problem. A local medical society, medical school, or accredited hospital may also be able to help you find a suitable doctor.

If your osteoporosis is especially advanced, your doctor may suggest you consult a rheumatologist or an orthopedic surgeon. A rheumatologist is a specialist in diseases of the muscles and skeleton, which include arthritis and other bone and joint problems (see page 81). The orthopedic surgeon is versed in preventing and repairing fractures (see page 82).

Into the Laboratory

In diagnosing your osteoporosis, your doctor will visually examine your back, hip, wrist, and limbs. He or she will ask you questions about your medical and family history. Your doctor may also conduct one or more of a number of the following laboratory tests or procedures.

Blood Tests

A blood test involves taking a small sample of your blood for analysis. Because calcium and other substances in your blood rise and fall in relation to what you consumed at your most recent meal, blood tests are usually taken in the morning after a twelve-hour fast.

Sometimes the procedure involves pricking the end of a finger and drawing off a small volume of blood. More often, blood is taken with a syringe and needle from a big vein on the front surface of your elbow. There are a large number of tests that can be conducted on the blood to indicate any number of things about its chemical and physical characteristics.

In most cases, blood tests will help your physician to determine whether your bone loss is the result of a disease other than osteoporosis.

BLOOD CHEMISTRY GROUP:　One key test your doctor is likely to do on the sample of blood that is collected is called a blood chemistry group test. This test may have any one of a variety of different commercial names, depending upon the laboratory conducting it. Typically, your blood will be tested for the presence and quantity of a number of chemicals.

The crucial ones for excluding other bone ailments are calcium and phosphorus. Too much calcium in your bloodstream suggests that your bones may not be using sufficient quantities of the mineral. Given that the typical osteoporosis patient is unlikely to have an imbalance of calcium in the bloodstream, the likely diagnosis is osteomalacia (page 12) rather than osteoporosis.

Another substance likely to be tested for in a blood chemistry group test is alkaline phosphatase, an enzyme involved in the use of calcium by the body. Too much of it would also suggest osteomalacia.

Yet another substance to be tested for in a blood chemistry workup will be creatinine, a chemical compound produced by your body's normal metabolism. This will help determine whether you have any kidney damage, which will be a factor in assessing the appropriateness of calcium supplementation and vitamin D administration. The creatinine test will inform your doctor as to how well the kidneys excrete waste products.

COMPLETE BLOOD COUNT:　Another common blood test done on patients suffering from any number of complaints is called the complete blood count (CBC). It tells the doctor whether you are anemic (that is, without enough red blood cells), leukopenic (that is, having too few white blood cells), or thrombocytopenic (that is, short of certain blood components called platelets or thrombocytes, which may be due to some medications). It may direct the doctor to conduct other tests as well.

ERYTHROCYTE SEDIMENTATION RATE: This special blood test measures the speed at which red blood cells fall to the bottom of a glass tube. In patients with widespread inflammation, the cells will fall rapidly through the serum, and the red blood cell sedimentation rate, familiarly known as the "sed rate," will be described as high. In good health, the cells only fall five or ten millimeters, and the result is termed a low or normal sed rate.

This test is useful in several circumstances. One is to eliminate the possibility that a type of cancer known as multiple myeloma is the cause of the bone wasting. Other conditions associated with osteoporosis and a high sed rate are rheumatoid arthritis and inflammatory bowel disease; in cases in which these diseases are very active, the development of osteoporosis is more rapid.

Urine Tests

Urinalysis involves a number of tests and may be useful in several ways, including the monitoring of the effect of certain drugs on the body. Protein and red blood cells in the urine are signs of kidney inflammation and may be the only ones since the process is almost always painless. If your doctor is trying to eliminate other possible causes of your bone loss, he or she will test to see how much calcium is leaving your body in your urine; high levels are consistent with osteoporosis.

As in the blood tests, your doctor may also be concerned with creatinine levels. Too high a ratio of creatinine to calcium suggests that calcium is being lost from the bones but that primary osteoporosis is not the cause.

X-rays

An x-ray is essentially a photograph, only the content of the photograph is the interior structure rather than the exterior appearance of the body part x-rayed. It is less complete than a photograph, permitting one to distinguish only areas where there are sharp contrasts in x-ray density, most particularly the bones. When an x-ray is taken, you will be positioned below the "camera" and asked to remain still for a moment while the film is exposed. The film will be developed in minutes.

While an x-ray film shows bone shape clearly, it is not as useful a tool as it might be in diagnosing and following the progression of osteoporosis. The bone loss is not a matter of the bones becoming smaller. Rather, they retain their shape but lose density. Not until 30 percent or more of the bone mass has been lost is the loss discernible in an x-ray.

One use of x-rays can be particularly useful in screening for osteoporosis. The jaw is often among the first of the bones to lose density. As a result, your dentist may well be in a position to see early warning signs of bone loss.

To further complicate matters, there is as yet no widely used system for assuring that x-rays taken over a period of years are comparable, given differences in exposure, equipment, and other factors.

RADIOGRAPHIC DENSITOMETRY: There is also a variation on traditional x-ray technology in which an x-ray "picture" is taken of the fingers and of a piece of aluminum alloy. Using the known density of the aluminum as the basis for comparison, a computer can then scan the bone and make a more accurate determination of the density of the bone.

Although this test is unable to distinguish between trabecular and cortical bone, it is useful in assessing the progression of the bone loss. This and other new ways of taking pictures of bone are often more useful than traditional x-rays (see Bone Scans, CT Scan, and Photon Absorptiometry, pages 43 and 44).

CT Scan

CT means "computed tomography" (it's also sometimes called computerized axial tomography or a CAT scan). It is often used in examining osteoporosis of the spinal column.

A CT scanner is an x-ray "camera" that is hooked up to a computer. A traditional x-ray machine takes a picture from only one angle, as a camera does. But a CT scan, thanks to the computer's presence, takes literally thousands of readings. The computer can then reassemble the images into one picture that represents a cross section of the body part(s) being studied. In short, by circling around the part of the body being "photographed," the CT scanner doesn't see it from one angle but sees all around it. The test takes roughly half an hour to complete.

CT can help your doctor to judge the condition of cortical and trabecular bone separately; since the latter is more likely to be lost in osteoporosis, this determination is valuable. The CT scan produces a "picture" that suggests a bone's density and is usually considered the best available method for determining early bone loss of the spine.

As with photon absorptiometry, CT scans are not perfect. There are no comparative standards for determining what is "normal" or to indicate relative bone loss to others of the same age, sex, and race. The CT also uses substantially more radiation than photon absorptiometry. The nature of the human skeleton is also a factor, as bone strength varies throughout the body, meaning that a test conducted in one site does not necessarily indicate bone loss elsewhere. In addition, two patients with the same degree of bone loss may have entirely different disease courses: one may have fractures, the other not.

Bone Scans

Nuclear or radioisotope scanning involves the use of small amounts of radioactive materials. Isotopes are administered and are absorbed by organs or other body parts (in this case, the bones) and then can be seen through the use of a special device that "scans" for the radioactivity. The picture that is produced can offer information about the condition of the bone being examined.

If your bone pain is limited to one localized area, your doctor may elect to perform a bone scan. This test involves the injection of a radioactive isotope. It takes about three hours for the isotope to reach the bone, and then about an hour for the scanner to take its "pictures."

The pictures will help the doctor identify fractures or unusual bone activity. The amount of radiation used is quite low, and your system will be free of it within hours.

Photon Absorptiometry

Photon absorptiometry is a kind of bone scan, but in this procedure the radioactive isotope is not put into the body but into a "source" or mechanical device that sends beams of radiation out for scanning. Absorptiometry equipment comes in two basic configurations.

SINGLE-PHOTON ABSORPTIOMETRY: This is the more commonly found variety of photon absorptiometry, and it is used to investigate the density of peripheral bones, like those in the leg or arm.

Single-photon absorptiometry functions by passing a beam from the source through the bone. A receiver then measures the strength of the signal that emerges on the other side. A strong signal means that less radiation has been absorbed by the bone, indicating that the bone has lost density and weakened. A weaker signal suggests that a stronger, healthier bone has absorbed more of the radiation. The time required for the single-photon absorptiometry test is about ten minutes.

The test is quite accurate. It measures losses of less than 3 percent of bone mass (in comparison with roughly 30 percent using traditional x-rays). However, the bone usually tested is the forearm, because the test requires that the soft tissues surrounding the bone being measured be of uniform thickness (meaning that the test will not accurately measure the density of bones in the hip or spine).

The loss of bone mass in the forearm usually approximates that lost from the spine, so this test is useful for screening for osteoporosis in older people. However, it is not of much value in following the progress of the disease in people already known to have suffered serious bone loss. A significant advantage of this test is that it requires less than 1 percent of the radiation of a traditional x-ray.

DUAL-PHOTON ABSORPTIOMETRY: In this variety of absorptiometry testing, better results are obtained in examining the spine and hip bones. In it, two beams of radiation at two different energy levels are sent through the bone. By measuring two levels of absorption, the distorting effects of different thicknesses of overlying soft tissue can be corrected for. The test takes approximately an hour to complete.

Despite its advantages, the test is not perfect. Deformed vertebrae and calcium deposits can distort the results, and neither single- nor dual-photon absorptiometry distinguish between cortical and trabecular bone.

In short, these tests are useful in helping to make general assessments of osteoporosis but are best used in conjunction with other determinations. Although special equipment like photon absorptiometry machines is new and expensive, it is quite widely available. (See also C T Scan, page 43.)

Biopsy

A small piece of tissue, called a biopsy, can be removed surgically and examined under a microscope. The procedure will probably involve the administration of a local anesthetic and will be over almost as soon as it begins. In osteoporosis, the most likely tissue for examination are sections of the rib and pelvic bones.

BONE BIOPSY: If your physician suspects that you have primary osteoporosis, he or she may propose a bone biopsy just to be sure. The bone biopsy will allow the doctor to rule out cancer as a possible cause for the weakening of your bones. It will also allow the doctor to learn about bone resorption and formation and to differentiate between osteomalacia and osteoporosis.

ENDOMETRIAL BIOPSY: If your doctor prescribes estrogen replacement therapy, he or she will be concerned if any abnormal menstrual bleeding occurs. If it does, the doctor may well advise an endometrial biopsy, in which a small piece of tissue from the lining of the uterus is removed and studied.

PAP SMEAR: A related test is called the Papanicolaou test or "Pap smear." Your doctor obtains a scraping of secretions from the cervix using a wooden spatula. The cells are then examined for indications of cervical cancers or other abnormalities. This test is a standard part of a gynecological examination and is especially important in women undergoing estrogen replacement therapy.

Medication

Some drugs have life-threatening interactions with other drugs, so be sure your physician knows not only what pills you are allergic to but also all the other drugs you are taking, especially if they were prescribed by another doctor. Bring your medications with you to your appointment if you have any doubts as to what they are or if you have trouble remembering their names or pill sizes.

Don't forget to mention any over-the-counter preparations you are taking, including antacids, cough syrups, constipation remedies, aspirin, and mineral or vitamin supplements. These and other generally available medications are also important to your body's chemistry.

If you are or become pregnant, you should discuss with your doctor the medications you are taking.

Be careful to follow the instructions you are given regarding dosage. Do not increase the number of tablets or capsules you take without your doctor's knowledge.

If you have ever had an allergic reaction to a drug, be sure to inform your doctor. It's the wrong drug for you, and your doctor needs to know that and to make the information a part of your medical records.

Generic vs. Brand Names

In reading about and discussing drugs, it is important to know the difference between generic and brand names. The generic name is the name a drug is given at its first discovery or concoction in a laboratory. It identifies the drug as being of a unique chemistry and different from all others. When that drug is marketed, however, it is given another name, a brand name.

When the Food and Drug Administration approves a drug for sale and use, generally one drug manufacturer has developed it and is licensed to sell it. The drug is then sold under a brand name, but with its generic name in smaller letters on the package as well. A number of years after its release, a drug becomes public property and other manufacturers can also sell it. At that point, there are likely to be a number of brand names under which the drug is sold. To make matters more complicated, some manufacturers may sell the drug under its own name as a generic and not give it a brand name. As a general rule, drugs sold as generics are less expensive than brand names.

In finding the drug or drugs your doctor prescribes for you in the following pages, look for it under its generic name; if you are unable to find a particular drug, look it up but be sure to check the index, where both brand and generic names are listed alphabetically. If you are unable to find the drug you are taking in these pages, there are a number of reference books cited in Chapter 5 to which you can go for further information about the medication (page 145).

Potential Side Effects

The potential side effects of drugs are extremely diverse. Some are trivial and transient, others permanent and profound. While a catalogue of the potential side effects of many drugs can be frightening, a little knowledge and understanding of them can go a long way toward alleviating much of the concern.

Your physician is by far your best guide through the complexity of potential untoward effects. He or she will discuss with you those that occur in as many as 3 to 5 percent of persons taking the drug in question. Your doctor may also deal with even rarer side effects simply because of their degree of danger.

This is a difficult area for both you and your doctor. On occasion, people who have been informed of a severe side effect that occurs in only one in a thousand patients will refuse to take that medication. In such cases, the physician often regrets this decision because his knowledge and judgment tell him that the medication in question will have a powerfully favorable effect on the patient. There is no substitute for complete openness and trust between the two persons in this delicate situation; each must honor the other's opinion.

To facilitate a more detailed discussion of the potential side effects of drugs that may be prescribed for you, we can assign letters to three grades of problems. "A" signifies those side effects that are present only while the medication is being taken; "B" indicates side effects that persist briefly after the medication is discontinued; and "C" indicates those that are permanent.

These side effect "grades" usually reflect the speed with which the drug is chemically destroyed or excreted by the body. Drugs like aspirin usually have only "A" effects, while estrogen therapies may have "B" or "C" effects.

The symptoms of drug toxicity can be classified into the following eight categories.

GENERAL: General side effects include swelling of the soft tissues with water retention (edema), fatigue, unexplained weight gain or loss, sweating, and fever. Generally these are "A" effects and not of great consequence, although fever may be a forerunner of more serious problems.

GASTROINTESTINAL: Abdominal pain, dyspepsia (indigestion), nausea and vomiting, gastritis (inflammation of the stomach lining), peptic ulcer, bleeding into the bowels, diarrhea, stomatitis (inflammation of the mouth), loss of appetite, and jaundice (liver disease with yellowing of the skin) are gastrointestinal side effects. Peptic ulcer, gastrointestinal bleeding, and jaundice are of concern despite being "A" effects. The sudden appearance of black or dark red stools signals gastrointestinal bleeding (dried blood may appear black rather than red in the stool) and is a medical emergency, possibly requiring immediate transfusion of blood. Jaundice may signal the onset of profound liver failure, and if it appears, all medication should be withdrawn.

SKIN: All manner of skin irritations ranging from hives to a measles-like rash can occur. Sometimes little red dots on the skin (the medical term is petechiae), easy bruising, itching, or decreased or increased growth of hair result from taking certain drugs.

NERVOUS SYSTEM: Symptoms in this category include headache, confusion, dizziness, deafness, a change in visual acuity, somnolence, and a ringing in the ears. Most of these are "A" side effects, but hearing and vision problems can be "C" side effects with some drugs.

RESPIRATORY SYSTEM: Asthma, bronchospasm, and pleurisy (inflammation of the membrane lining the lungs) can occur.

HEMATOPOIETIC SYSTEM: The tissues of the body where blood cells are manufactured, the bone marrow and lymph nodes, are referred to as the hematopoietic system. "B" and "C" side effects can occur and are of concern. With some drugs, repeated blood counts are obtained to detect the appearance of such problems as aplastic anemia (in which no red cells are being made), agranulocytosis (when the number of granulocytes or polys, white blood cells that fight infection, decreases radically), and thrombocytopenia (reduced number of platelets). These are dreaded complications, and most drugs capable of causing them are kept out of our drugstores and are not available for purchase. That may not be so, however, in countries with less stringent laws.

UROGENITAL SYSTEM: Nephritis (inflammation of the kidneys), cystitis (inflammation of the urinary bladder), bloody urine, or damaged eggs or sperm may occur and may be "A," "B," or "C" side effects.

INDUCTION OF CANCER: The greatest danger of estrogen replacement therapy is the possibility of cancer of the lining of the uterus, called the endometrium. While it is difficult to tell what the probability is of a typical patient developing this "C"-type hazard, it is true that the concerns are usually dealt with successfully if detected early. Any bleeding that is abnormal in timing or quantity is an indication, as the doctors call it, for immediate examination, Pap smears, and perhaps an endometrial biopsy.

An important reason for looking over the preceding list is to encourage you to be watchful. Any of these indications (or other changes or discomforts not cited here) should be reported to your physician immediately upon their appearance. Your doctor may not change your drug program, but when armed with complete knowledge of your condition, he or she is certainly in a better position to advise you.

Analgesics

ACETAMINOPHEN
Prescribed For: Osteoporotic pain.
Effect: The reduction of mild to moderate pain.
Dosage: 500 to 1,000 mg every four hours for pain.
Symptom Relief: Within thirty minutes of ingestion.
Side Effects: Minor skin rash, drowsiness, or abnormal bruising or bleeding may occur, but generally only in long-term users.
Brand Names: Acetaminophen is available without a prescription, though in some combinations with other drugs a prescription is required (see Codeine, page 52.) Among the brand names under which this drug is sold are Datril, Tylenol, and Excedrin.

ASPIRIN
Prescribed For: Pain involved in the muscles and bones as a result of osteoporotic fractures.

What we have come to refer to as aspirin in conversation is also known by the chemical name acetylsalicylic acid or ASA. As this name suggests, aspirin is a member of the salicylate family, drugs which the body breaks down into salicylate, a chemical found in willow tree bark and other plants. Although the favorable effects of the bark were known to some of our remote ancestors, the responsible chemical was not identified or made until early in this century. The compounds relieve mild to moderate pain and the redness and swelling of inflammation.

Effects: Reduction of pain and inflammation.

Dosage: 300 to 600 mg every six hours for pain.

Side Effects: Gastrointestinal distress, signaled by indigestion, nausea, vomiting, and stomach irritation; take with meals or milk to reduce such discomforts. A comforting feature of aspirin is that because it has been on the market for so long, its side effects are well known. The same cannot be said for more recently introduced agents.

Aspirin causes some people to bruise easily and can interfere with the blood's ability to clot, which is why it is occasionally given to prevent heart attacks due to blood clots in the coronary arteries. If you tend to bleed easily, aspirin may not be the best choice of treatment for you.

Brand Names: Bayer, Ecotrin, Empirin, buffered aspirin, and numerous others.

Aspirin comes in tablets, capsules, and liquid forms. Some varieties are buffered, that is, treated with an antacid to prevent in part irritation of the lining of the stomach. Some preparations release the salicylate into your system slowly, over a period of hours. Follow your doctor's recommendations in selecting a brand suitable to your needs.

(Note: There are innumerable "house brands" available, in which the generic drug is sold under the name of the store or chain selling it. The ASA molecule itself is identical in all brands. The various pills into which it is compounded, however, are put together in different ways. One test you can do is to drop an aspirin into water: if it disintegrates swiftly, forming a cloudy solution in the water, it is probably easier on your stomach than one that remains relatively intact when submerged.

CODEINE

Prescribed For: Codeine is a painkiller, a mild narcotic drug derived from opium.

Effect: A very effective analgesic that relieves moderate to severe pain, codeine is also used to control cough and diarrhea. In the control of pain, it is useful to take another analgesic, such as acetaminophen or aspirin, with codeine.

Dosage: Varies greatly with preparation used.

Side Effects: Because codeine is a narcotic and, consequently, addictive, it is generally used only in short-term therapy.

In addition to concerns about its being addicting, you should be aware that its potential side effects include such gastrointestinal problems as nausea, vomiting, and loss of appetite, dry mouth, trouble urinating, and constipation. Constipation, in particular, can be a problem for older patients.

Codeine may also induce drowsiness, dizziness, or sleepiness, so avoid driving or operating machinery when taking this drug.

Brand Names: Codeine is sold in the United States only as a prescription drug. Codeine phosphate with acetaminophen is sold under the brand names Aceta with Codeine, Amahen with Codeine, Anacin-3 with Codeine, Bancap with Codeine, Capital with Codeine, Codalan, Codap, Empracet with Codeine, G-2, G-3, Maxigesic, Panadol with Codeine, Phenaphen with Codeine, Proval No. 3, Tega-Code-M, Tylenol with Codeine, and Ty-Tab. Codeine phosphate and codeine sulfate are sold with aspirin as Anexsia with Codeine, A.S.A. & Codeine Compound, Ascriptin with Codeine, Buff-A Comp, Bufferin with Codeine, Emcodeine Tablets, Empirin with Codeine, and Fiorinal with Codeine.

Oxycodone hydrochloride is a related drug with similar uses and potential side effects. Oxycodone hydrochloride with acetaminophen is sold as Percocet and Tylox. Oxycodone hydrochloride with aspirin bears the brand names Codoxy and Percodan.

OTHER ANALGESICS

Although as yet not proven conclusively to be of benefit in treating osteoporotic pain, diflunisal, fenprofen, ibuprofen, indomethacin, meclofenamate, naproxen, piroxicam, sulindac, and tolmetin are other analgesics that are occasionally used in its treatment.

Fluoride Therapy

It has been observed that postmenopausal women who grew up in areas where the fluoride content of the water is above average are less likely to experience vertebral fractures. This has led to experiments in the use of sodium fluoride.

Sodium fluoride stimulates bone cells to increase bone formation by increasing the number of osteoblasts (bone-forming cells) and the deposition of new bone matrix. Some preliminary trials have found that, when given with calcium supplements, sodium fluoride significantly decreases the occurrence of vertebral fractures. However, the frequent side effects (stomach upset and rheumatic symptoms in the legs and feet) and the unproven nature of the treatment make it still experimental—it does not yet have U.S. Food and Drug Administration approval for general use. You may wish to discuss the possibility of fluoride therapy with your doctor, as it may be approved shortly or there may be a medical center nearby conducting experiments with it. It may be useful in treating you in the years immediately following menopause.

In general, this therapy is reserved for severe cases of osteoporosis. It is generally prescribed in conjunction with calcium supplements and vitamin D, though in some cases it may be used with estrogen replacement therapy (page 54).

FLUORIDE

Prescribed For: Severe osteoporosis.

Effect: Decreases calcium resorption from bones and increases calcium deposition, thereby helping to restore skeletal mass.

Dosage: 40 to 65 mg daily in conjunction with calcium and vitamin D supplements or with estrogens.

Symptom Relief: Decreases incidence of vertebral fractures.
Side Effects: Nearly one in two patients taking full-dose fluoride
supplements experience pain in the knees and ankles, vomiting,
or anemia.

Hormone Therapy

Estrogens are female hormones, androgens male hormones.
Both have applications in treating osteoporosis.

Estrogens are produced by the ovaries, and menopause signals
the end of their production. As discussed in Chapter 1, this leads
to a rapid demineralization of the bones as the estrogen, which
limits the resorption of calcium from the bones, ceases to do so.

Estrogen replacement therapy (ERT) usually involves a four-
week schedule of medication: three weeks of daily doses of
estrogen followed by a week without. The reappearance of menstrual bleeding is secondary to withdrawal of estrogen. The hormone builds up the lining of the uterus (endometrium) and its
withdrawal produces endometrial shedding.

You should observe carefully the bleeding that occurs while
undergoing ERT. Timely menstrual bleeding is to be expected,
but any other vaginal bleeding should be brought to your doctor's attention immediately. Your doctor will probably then perform an endometrial biopsy to establish the nature of the bleeding.
In any case, the use of estrogens calls for pelvic and breast examinations at roughly six-month intervals. Pap smears should
also be a standard part of the monitoring process. (See page 39
for discussion of these and other laboratory tests.)

Estrogen in itself will not produce an increase in bone mass.
In fact, in addition to limiting the withdrawal of calcium from
the bones, estrogen functionally limits the calcium deposited. As
a result, estrogen's principal value is not as a cure for bone loss
but to slow the loss during the postmenopausal phase when it
is likely to be the greatest. There is also some evidence that rate
of fractures in osteoporosis sufferers decreases after ERT therapy.

The greatest risk with ERT is in the incidence of endometrial cancer. While the occurrence of this form of cancer is roughly one in one thousand in the general population, there is a sixfold increase in the risk in those who undergo ERT for a period of less than five years; the danger is fifteen times greater among women who take estrogen for longer periods. While endometrial cancer is not difficult to detect, rarely fatal, and treatments for it generally available, the risk of developing cancer must be balanced with the possible benefits of estrogen therapy.

These risks are usually assessed on the basis of age. In elderly women whose bone mass has already been significantly reduced, the long-term use of estrogens is generally thought to be inappropriate: the cancer-causing properties of estrogen make it dangerous, and its effectiveness in such patients has yet to be clearly demonstrated. On the other hand, the use of estrogen replacement therapy in younger women who have had their ovaries removed or who are in the early stages of menopause can be an appropriate therapy.

Estrogen has another incidental benefit: it provides some protection against heart disease. Estrogen apparently increases blood levels of one of the types of cholesterol, high-density lipoprotein (HDL), and lowers blood levels of the other, low-density lipoprotein (LDL). HDL is regarded as the "good cholesterol," since a higher ratio of HDL to LDL is associated with a decrease in the risk of arteriosclerosis, commonly referred to as hardening of the arteries.

To use it or not to use it? Estrogen replacement therapy is not to be used without due deliberation. An assessment must be made of its attendant risks and benefits. In women who enter menopause prematurely, in particular when the cause is the surgical removal of the ovaries, the risk of osteoporosis is thought to be particularly high; in such cases the use of ERT is often warranted.

In other cases, the decision may be made on the basis of the other risk factors for osteoporosis cited in Chapter 1 (page 13, "Am I at Risk?"). If you are, for example, very slight, smoke heavily, consume few calcium-rich foods, and lead a largely sedentary life, you are likely to be an excellent candidate for ERT; on the other hand, if you have a large frame, love dairy foods more than anything in life, and perform demanding physical labor daily, your physician may well advise against ERT during your menopause years. If you have a history of blood clots, active liver disease, or have had breast or endometrial cancer, some other approach is likely to be better.

In order to limit the risk of cancer, another hormone, progestin, is often prescribed in tandem with the estrogen (in such cases, doctors often term it hormone replacement therapy, or HRT). The progestin is taken during the last week or so of the cyclical HRT, and it serves to protect the lining of the uterus from being overstimulated by the estrogen. There is also some evidence that suggests that an ample calcium intake (1,500 milligrams daily) and frequent exercise may allow the required dose of estrogen to be reduced.

HRT in any of its forms is not appropriate for all women going through menopause. On balance, the benefits and risks argue for only carefully considered use of this therapy. One sensible use, as expressed by the 1984 Consensus Development Conference on Osteoporosis that was sponsored by the National Institutes of Health, is for its prescription for women whose ovaries are removed before age fifty, since they are at especially high risk of osteoporosis. Another group of candidates are women who have passed through a natural menopause but who have multiple risk factors.

Androgens are the male hormones responsible for the development of male characteristics. Testosterone and androsterone are androgens. They also decrease the excretion of calcium and lead to an increased muscle mass, stimulating their abuse by athletes trying to add bulk and strength.

Some synthetic androgens decrease bone loss in postmenopausal women. Although studies of the long-term effects are not yet complete, it appears that these drugs may be a valuable alternative to estrogen therapy. The androgens can have undesirable side effects—male characteristics can result from their use, like an increase in body hair and a deepening of the voice—but these effects can be minimized by using them, like estrogen, on a three-weeks-on, one-week-off basis.

ESTROGEN

Prescribed For: Preventing and limiting further loss of bone mass.

Effect: The withdrawal of calcium from the bones is decreased by the estrogens; hot flushes are less frequent and less severe; vaginal dryness and discomfort may be relieved.

Dosage: .625 to 1.25 mg of estrogen compounds or 50 micrograms of ethinyl estradiol; may be taken in pill form or as a cream or ointment for application to the vagina, in some cases as a skin patch; usually taken daily for a period of three weeks then withdrawn one week; treatment may last several years or even longer.

Side Effects: Menstrual bleeding will occur during the one-week break between doses; the risk of endometrial cancer is increased considerably (page 50); some patients report swelling of the breasts, nausea, high blood pressure, edema (fluid retention), headaches, or weight gain.

ANDROGENS

Prescribed For: Reduction of bone loss in postmenopausal women.

Effect: Androgens are anabolic hormones, ones that build up body mass and protein (as contrasted to catabolic hormones, like adrenal corticosteroids, which destroy protein and reduce muscle mass). The precise effects of androgens on bones are unknown, but they are thought to reduce bone turnover and produce a modest increase in total body calcium.

Dosage: 2 to 6 mg daily for three weeks; one week off.

Side Effects: May induce certain male characteristics, including muscle development and hair growth; acne also occurs in some patients, as well as a deepening of the voice; may also cause changes in blood lipoproteins, favoring the development of atherosclerosis or the fatty deterioration of artery walls; these effects have greatly reduced the use of androgens in treating osteoporosis.

Brand Name: Winstrol

Vitamin D Supplements

You are less likely to require vitamin D supplementation than calcium supplements: while this vitamin is critical to your body being able to absorb calcium, getting enough of it is not the problem that sufficient calcium is.

The Recommended Dietary Allowance for vitamin D is 400 international units per day. There are some dietary sources like fatty fish (herring, salmon, sardines, and tuna), egg yolks, and milk (which in its natural state has little vitamin D but in commercial processing is fortified with the vitamin), but the larger portion of the average person's vitamin D comes from the sun, which stimulates its formation in the skin.

If you eat a balanced diet and are exposed to the sun daily for some time (some experts place the time required between fifteen and sixty minutes), the chances are that your body manufactures enough vitamin D for your needs. However, if you consume few foods containing the vitamin and you are housebound or by custom are heavily clothed or if air pollution is a constant problem in your area, you might be well advised to take one of the many generally available multivitamin supplements.

Read the label on the multivitamin to be sure the preparation contains the recommended 400 international units of vitamin D. It is not necessary to take more than 400 units, as too much of the vitamin can stimulate bone loss. Thus, according to the American Society for Bone and Mineral Research, you should avoid taking more than 1,000 international units a day.

Pregnant women in particular should be alert to their intake of vitamin D. Too little vitamin D can lead to fetal abnormalities, but pregnant women are at high risk of kidney damage from large amounts. Consume enough but not too much: the suitable range is not less than 400 but not more than 800 international units.

It is downright dangerous to take very large doses, as too much can result in a well-recognized syndrome called, reasonably enough, hypervitaminosis D. This state is characterized by calcium deposition in many parts of the body where it should not be. Among other effects are kidney troubles, as the excess calcium can cause a decline of function and kidney failure.

Other Medications

CALCITONIN: The hormone calcitonin is referred to as an anti-hypercalcemic factor, as it reduces the removal of calcium from the bones when the blood calcium level goes up (page 9). Its release is stimulated by too much calcium in the blood.

In Europe, synthetic calcitonin has been used extensively as a treatment for osteoporosis. Given by injection, the calcitonin has been shown to instigate observable increases in bone mass. However, it appears the effect is temporary, and that within twelve months, despite continuing injections, the benefit ceases.

There are also ongoing experiments in the United States involving the use of a combination of calcitonin and phosphate. In both cases, the body's natural calcitonin, produced by the thyroid gland, is supplemented by synthetic calcitonin. Studies are continuing, so calcitonin may prove to be a viable treatment for osteoporosis.

It is used very successfully in a condition called Paget's disease of bone, in which bone metabolism is greatly accelerated in patches of bone here and there in the skeleton.

Dosage: 100 international units per day by injection.

Side Effects: Allergic reactions to the injection after several consecutive doses.

Brand Name: Calcimar.

PARATHORMONE: Another area of experimentation involves use of a synthesized portion of parathormone, the calcium-regulating hormone of the parathyroid gland (page 9).

In the spontaneous illness called hyperparathyroidism (in which too much parathormone is produced), bone loss occurs and the blood calcium level becomes elevated. These findings are the opposite of what is needed in the treatment of osteoporosis. Paradoxically, however, there is some evidence that administration of the synthesized fragment of the hormone in small doses causes an increase in the trabecular bone mass. Such preliminary studies need confirmation before the hormone can be recommended for treatment. When (or if) it is approved, it will almost certainly be at a low dose and in combination with other agents.

DRUG COMBINATIONS: Although each is listed separately, we have mentioned several possible combinations of medications. Actually, it is very uncommon to take only one medication for severe osteoporosis. There has been much study of various combinations; these have disclosed effects which were unexpectedly different from the effects of the individual drugs.

Another approach has been to use drugs intermittently. This may prevent tachyphylaxis, or loss of drug effect, ascribed to the body changing in response to the drug and becoming resistant to it. Some programs are designed to "turn on" the osteoblasts using certain drugs, stimulating the bone cells to lay down matrix and calcium, and then suddenly convert to other drugs which will "turn off" the osteoclasts and thus prevent bone removal. The cycle is repeated over and over.

The most common combination these days is estrogen and calcium. It is impossible to predict what new combinations of drugs current and future research efforts will show to be effective.

Calcium Supplements

Vitamin and mineral supplements are not the panacea that the thousands of claims made for them would suggest. They don't cure arthritis or cancer, they can't guarantee youth or longevity, they may or may not have a particular benefit in treating the common cold. Yet in some situations supplements have been shown to be of definite importance; in others, there is enough evidence to suggest that they might be useful enough to argue for their consumption.

Calcium supplementation makes sense on the latter grounds. We know the single most important mineral to the patient with osteoporosis is calcium—by now, that surely comes as no shock to you. So it is hardly surprising that some research suggests that calcium supplementation is linked with a decrease in vertebral fractures. Other data indicate that the more calcium that is consumed, the more that is absorbed in most patients.

This latter finding is all the more important when coupled with the fact that in order to consume the Recommended Dietary Allowances of calcium, many people, women in particular, would have to eat a great many more calories than is their wont. After all, even two glasses of milk plus a cup of yogurt plus a one ounce serving of cheese amounts to only 1,000 milligrams of calcium, fully a third short of the 1,500 some experts recommend for post-menopausal women. Unless you have an inordinate taste for milk and dairy products, supplements may make sense for you.

However, if your doctor recommends that you begin estrogen replacement therapy, don't try and convince him that calcium supplements are as efficient in helping to restore bone mass. Estrogen replacement therapy (page 37) is, for certain patients at certain times, the best way of treating bone loss. Calcium may help as well, either in conjunction with estrogen replacement therapy or on its own. But the consensus of recent research has it that calcium supplementation is not to be regarded as a substitute for estrogen replacement therapy in the years following menopause.

How Much Calcium Do You Get?

But first things first. In order to determine whether your diet contains sufficient calcium, consult the table (page 63) for the Recommended Dietary Allowances for calcium. That will tell you what you should be consuming.

Now, consult the table (page 101) of foods rich in calcium. For the next week, record all the calcium-rich foods you eat; at the end of that time, divide the total number of milligrams of calcium you have consumed by the number of days. Where do you stand?

The chances are very good that you will find that your intake of calcium is well less than the recommended levels. Again, the average American woman consumes only 450 milligrams of calcium daily—and that simply isn't enough.

You have two choices. You can increase your intake of calcium from dietary sources. Thus, you might drink more milk and eat more dairy products, unboned fish (canned salmon and sardines), and leafy green vegetables (in particular, cabbage, collard greens, kale, and mustard and turnip greens). (For a detailed discussion of nutritional strategies for increasing calcium intake, see Chapter 4, page 100.)

However, one recent study found that the administration of calcium as milk or as capsules containing such salts as calcium carbonate or calcium acetate resulted in the absorption of the same amount of calcium. It would appear that there is nothing magic about the milk or the pills. So if reaching the 1,500 milligrams recommended for postmenopausal women simply isn't possible relying on dietary sources, supplementation is your next choice. It may be your best option, especially if you are lactose intolerant, that is, if you have difficulty digesting milk products (page 102).

Opting for calcium supplements, however, is a choice to be made only after incorporating as many dietary sources of calcium as possible. But for some, it may be the only way to reach the recommended levels of calcium consumption.

The verdict is not yet in on the value of supplementation. Some scientists say it's important; others say its value is, at best, unproven. There seems general agreement that it is of evident value when taken in conjunction with estrogen replacement therapy; there is also evidence that supplements taken by postmenopausal women retard the loss of cortical bone. But as for premenopausal women and trabecular bone, the debate continues.

On the other hand, the only evidence that calcium supplements are harmful in any way is that in people who take massive amounts (more than 2,000 milligrams a day), kidney problems can develop, especially in persons with a history of kidney stones or "weak kidneys." Too much calcium may also limit to some degree your body absorption of other important minerals, including zinc, copper, iron, and magnesium. In any case, be sure to discuss the effect of supplementation with your physician. (If you are pregnant or lactating, having that discussion is especially pertinent. You must consume sufficient calcium to meet not only your own needs but those of your child as well.)

The fact is that taking a calcium supplement isn't difficult or

CALCIUM: THE RECOMMENDED DAILY ALLOWANCES

Infants up to 6 months	360 mg†
Infants 6 to 12 months	540 mg†
Children 1 to 10 years*	800 mg†
Adolescents 11 to 18 years	1,200 mg†
Pregnant/lactating women	1,600 mg†
Premenopausal women	1,000 mg^
Estrogen-treated women	1,000 mg^
Postmenopausal women	1,500 mg^
Men	1,000 mg^

* Weighing up to 62 pounds and standing no more than 52 inches tall
†Source: Recommended Dietary Allowances, 9th ed., Food and Nutrition Board of the National Academy of Sciences/National Research Council, 1980
^Source: 1984 National Institutes of Health Consensus Development Conference on Osteoporosis

Note: There has been much debate about the RDAs for calcium. Although the National Academy has yet to raise the recommended levels above the 800 mg level for postmenopausal and premenopausal women who are not pregnant, there is an emerging consensus for higher amounts like those cited by the NIH Conference.

expensive. You don't need a doctor's prescription, and calcium supplements are generally available at reasonable prices. They come in tablet, capsule, liquid, and powdered form. Certain brands of orange juice and cocoa and other products can be purchased that have been fortified with extra calcium. Some supplements come combined with vitamin D or other minerals, like magnesium. In general, however, it is advisable to avoid vitamin D supplements unless your doctor specifically recommends them.

Though they are available over the counter, calcium supplements, like any medication, are to be used with care. A sensible dosage for postmenopausal women is approximately 1,000 milligrams. That amount, in combination with a typical dietary intake of 500 milligrams of calcium, brings the daily sum to the recommended level of 1,500 milligrams. For premenopausal women, a 500 milligram supplement is recommended.

What Varieties of Calcium Supplements Are Available?

Not all supplements are the same. Some, according to a recent University of Maryland study, take so long to disintegrate in your gastrointestinal tract that they are poorly absorbed and of little value. It is also true that not all supplements share the same chemical makeup: calcium is combined with other substances to form calcium lactate, calcium gluconate, calcium carbonate, and others.

Until recently, calcium pills were about the size of a quarter; up to six or more a day were required to get the necessary calcium. Now, however, smaller, more convenient pills are generally available.

One relatively inexpensive source of supplementation is calcium carbonate. In order to get 1,000 milligrams of calcium, you need to take 2.5 grams of calcium carbonate. For maximum absorption, one 1,250 milligram tablet should be taken at midmorning, another at bedtime. Tums antacids are one sensible and inexpensive choice: one tablet contains 200 milligrams of calcium, so five per day will provide you with 1,000 milligrams.

Calcium carbonate is usually the cheapest of the calcium supplements. However, some people find calcium carbonate difficult to absorb, especially those with a low production of stomach acid. In other people, constipation is an unpleasant side effect. If this problem occurs, switch to a supplement that contains magnesium along with the calcium.

Calcium lactate is another candidate for supplementation, though it is not an option for those who are lactose intolerant (page 102). Often it is available in 650 milligram tablets, but because the calcium content of each tablet is low, twelve tablets per day are needed to obtain 1,000 milligrams of calcium. Other possibilities are calcium chloride (it tends to irritate some people's stomachs but is recommended for pickling instead of table salt) and calcium gluconate (like calcium lactate, its calcium content is relatively low, requiring that eleven 975 milligram tablets be taken daily; some people also find it too sweet). Another possibility is calcium levulinate, but it, too, has a very small amount of calcium per tablet and a strong taste (it tends to be salty and bitter).

Some other sources of calcium such as dolomite (a rock mineral) and bone meal may contain lead. Lead is a particular risk to children and women of childbearing age, and perhaps to the elderly as well. As a result, the FDA has issued a warning regarding the use of dolomite and bone meal for supplements. Avoid them.

Another point to remember is to take your supplement with fruit juice. Both its acid and vitamin C content will aid absorption.

Surgery

Almost without exception, surgical intervention directed toward the relief of osteoporosis is of an orthopedic nature, that is, a matter of repairing fractures. The notable exception is in treating people with unusual causes for osteoporosis, such as Cushing's syndrome. In such cases, there is an occasional need for endocrine surgery, but such treatments would be handled the same way as in the event the ailment (in our example, Cushing's syndrome) was not accompanied by osteoporosis.

Thus, we will be concerned with fractures in the following pages.

What Surgical Procedures Are Performed?

The four most common fractures in people with weakened bones are fractures of the hip, wrist, shoulder, and vertebrae. Even though the repair of some of these may not require an operation, your orthopedic surgeon is still the person to see. Much of his or her training is concerned with helping patients deal with the results of skeletal trauma.

WRIST FRACTURE: The wrist fracture, often called a Colles fracture, actually involves the wide part of the radius bone at the wrist joint (the radius is the larger bone that comes down to the thumb side of the hand). The exact nature of your break will determine for your doctor the mode of support, immobilization, or traction required. Usually, the bone can be returned to its proper position and be put into a splint of plaster of paris. This is done under anesthesia.

HIP FRACTURE: The broken hip involves the upper end of the femoral bone of the thigh. The upper end of the femur narrows as it approaches the hip joint (the "neck") and then increases in size at the hip joint itself to the ball-shaped extremity of the bone (the "head") that fits neatly into a socket-like concavity in the pelvic structure. The femur may break at the head, neck, or lower down between two major muscle attachment sites. Different treatment considerations arise in each of these, but all of them require open surgery under general anesthesia.

Treatment modes in the hip are changing. Internal fixation, as it is often called, is achieved by wires or screws put through the neck and inside the ball-shaped head. The slang description is "nailing the hip." Sometimes the "nail" is held by a metal plate which is firmly fastened to the outside of the straight upper portion of the bone.

If there is any sign of preexisting hip disease, such as arthritis, the surgeon may decide to carry the surgery a step further and replace the ball with a metal ball whose supporting arm is put into the inside, marrow space of the femur. Another possibility is total hip arthroplasty (or replacement), in which both sides of the joint are replaced with the insertion of a new socket and ball. Many of the modern methods allow you to stand and bear weight very soon after the operation, an important matter for elderly persons with severe osteoporosis.

The immediate results are impressive. People whose hip bones were badly deteriorated by osteoporosis or shattered in a fall often walk out of the hospital free of pain.

How long the prostheses (or "mechanical parts") will last is not yet known, as these operations are relatively new. However, those done to date seem to hold up well in moderate use and will certainly serve the elderly as long as required.

UPPER ARM FRACTURE: The head of the humerus or upper arm bone can also be broken in falls. Usually fractures of the humeral head are treated without an operation but with a cast. In some cases, various replacement procedures are performed.

VERTEBRAL FRACTURE: The very familiar crush fracture of the anterior portion of the vertebrae actually gets very little treatment except for pain control medication and the "tincture of time." Typically the pain begins to recede fairly promptly and is gone within two or three months. You end up just a bit shorter and a bit more bent over, but these changes will not impair your activities.

Sometimes if the pain persists and particularly if it is brought on by motion, a brace or a corset is prepared. (See Orthotics, page 126.) These are often uncomfortable, and many of them seem to spend more time in closets than on people's backs. In any case, their use is much in debate, as braces and corsets take some of the weight and muscle pull off your bones, thus depriving you of some portion of the biggest bone builder of all.

The Recovery

If you require an operation, your orthopedic surgeon will perform it, but its success depends heavily on you. Surgery to correct a fracture will not cure or eliminate the problem of bones weakened by osteoporosis. It is a treatment that, along with physical therapy and perhaps some medication, can help you in your fight against osteoporosis. In the event your surgery involves correcting a fracture, you must plan on investing time, energy, and effort together with some pain and discomfort in strengthening and exercising the surgically corrected bones. The muscles about the break operated upon may be underutilized, weak, and atrophied. Once the possibility of reasonable motion is restored, you can see that you will need to restore the muscles.

Physical Therapy

For many concerned with osteoporosis, the line between exercise and physical therapy is difficult to draw. After a fractured vertebra, supervised exercise like riding a stationary bicycle or swimming are often recommended for strengthening the back muscles. One could, therefore, distinguish between that sort of exercise program (calling it "physical therapy") and the exercise a young woman might do to develop her muscles and bones to avoid osteoporosis later. So when is exercise physical therapy and when is it exercise?

For convenience, let's say that physical therapy is the programmed approach to movement your doctor, physical therapist, or physiatrist prescribes (see pages 83 and 84 for discussion of the role of physical therapist and physiatrist). Usually physical therapy is, as its name suggests, part of a therapeutic program designed to help someone recover from an injury or surgery.

Every bit as important to the good health of your skeleton—whether you know you have osteoporosis now or whether your concern is with your body twenty years hence—is the pattern of continuing physical activity you should strive to establish to help your bones. In the case of a patient recovering, this activity should continue long after leaving the hospital and the appointments with the physical therapist have decreased in frequency.

In this chapter, the emphasis is on the care and treatment the medical professional can offer you after you have suffered bone loss and are at risk of—or have already experienced—osteoporotic fractures. Thus, we will talk about physical therapy in these pages. However, for a more general discussion of physical activity, see Chapter 4, "Self-Help," page 110. There the emphasis is on establishing a regime of regular exercise to minimize bone loss, both for those with osteoporosis and for others concerned about its risk in the coming years.

Weight-bearing Exercise

The space program has taught us about a great many things, including our bones.

During the Gemini missions, scientists monitored the astronauts' bones. What they observed is of particular interest to patients with osteoporosis. While weightless in space, the astronauts experienced small but significant losses in bone mass. Since all were young men and none were, obviously, menopausal, the loss of calcium from the bones was remarkable. The moral of this story is applicable to you: essential to bone strengthening is weight-bearing physical activity—something the astronauts simply couldn't get in space.

This doesn't translate into a quick trip to the local sports shop for you to buy a full array of barbells in order to fight osteoporosis. What it means is the more you carry yourself around, and the more vigorously you do it (and, therefore, the more weight-bearing exercise you get), the more good you will do your bones.

Exercise to the patient with osteoporosis is a matter of both recovery and maintenance. After a fracture, you need to strengthen the muscles that have weakened from disuse. There is also substantial evidence that exercise is the only way to significantly add to your bone mass, both in the vicinity of the break and elsewhere.

To some osteoporosis patients, recovery is largely a matter of physical activity. If your osteoporosis is the result of simple immobilization (as is the case with disuse osteoporosis, the variety suffered by, among others, people who are bedridden for long periods of time), then mobilization of the wasted bones and adjacent musculature may well be sufficient to promote a rapid cure.

On the other hand, if your problem is primary osteoporosis, of either the postmenopausal or senile varieties, you will need a full program of dietary strategies and perhaps medication as well.

Stay Active

Modest increases in weight-bearing activity can preserve bone mass, even in frail, elderly men and women. That's why maintaining an active lifestyle, walking rather than riding, climbing stairs instead of taking elevators, standing rather than sitting, can significantly lower the risk of developing osteoporosis. In the osteoporosis sufferer, further bone loss can be limited by a therapeutic program that includes sensible weight-bearing exercise.

It is thought that it is the bearing of the weight, which places actual physical stress on the bones, that cause the bones to respond by becoming bigger and stronger (this explains why, conversely, the astronauts in a state of weightlessness lost calcium from their bones). Exercise also increases blood flow to the bones, thereby increasing the available bone-building nutrients. Further, exercise generates mini-electrical currents within the bones that stimulate bone growth. Finally, exercise alters the hormonal balance, favoring those hormones which protect the bones.

The goal of physical therapy for the osteoporosis patient is simple: flexibility and strength are to be maintained or restored but with careful regard for the weakened bones, as they must be protected against further damage. Particularly if you have sustained any osteoporotic fractures, the kind, number, and intensity of your exercises must be determined by your medical advisors in order to meet your particular needs and work within the limitations imposed by your weakened frame. More than likely, your exercises will consist at least in part of weight-bearing exercise.

Your exercise must be part of your daily routine to be effective. The therapist cannot do it, but you must. This may require a big effort on your part. It may seem easier to stop than to continue with the exercises (they may seem difficult, even painful, or you may not feel as if you are getting better), but you must stay with them. Improving the stiffness or weakness that can accompany osteoporosis can take time, but following a program will, in the long term, help you in your battle.

That is not to say your daily exercises should be all pain and discomfort. In fact, if they are more than slightly painful, discuss your regimen with your doctor or physical therapist.

In some cases, one or more weekly trips to your physical therapist's office are part of the routine. In virtually all cases, it is the prescribed exercises done at home which are critical.

Unfortunately, no one else can do exercises for you. Others can sometimes help and so can special equipment, but, for the most part, exercises must be a part of the daily routine, done wherever you are with whatever is at hand.

Protect Your Bones

If you have osteoporosis, one of the most important pieces of advice you should give yourself every day is: "Be careful."

You shouldn't let your life come to a sudden stop, nor should you be afraid to go about living it. At the same time, however, as an osteoporosis sufferer you must learn a new set of "being-careful skills."

When a child learns to cross the street, he or she is given a few commonsense rules starting with "Stop, look, and listen" and "Be sure to look both ways." You must apply the same level of care and consideration.

Some safeguards are obvious. If you wear glasses for activities other than reading, wear them when you walk around the house. Avoid using ladders and standing on chairs to reach highly placed objects—get somebody else to change your lightbulbs, and re-arrange your closets so you aren't always climbing up to reach that warm sweater. If you use a cane, employ it around the house, too. Falls at home can be just as harmful as those in the outside world.

If you have sustained a fracture from a fall—or even if you simply have experienced a fall without breaking any bones—your doctor may thoroughly evaluate you. If you are worried that your balance is unsteady, ask your doctor about it.

Your doctor's evaluation means checking not only your medication—is it making you drowsy?—and your vision and hearing but also your physical condition. Your doctor may ask to observe you as you make such movements as rising from a chair, turning around, moving your head up-and-down and side-to-side, bending over, sitting, and performing other normal, day-to-day motions. He or she will be trying to establish that you are steady on your feet and that your sense of balance is sound.

Your doctor may go a step further in determining if there are hazards in your home or workplace that are just waiting to threaten the health of your bones. He or she may arrange for an occupational therapist to visit your home to search out any environmental hazards you may have overlooked, to recommend assistive devices if necessary (in some cases, a specific type of cane is in order, for example), and to instruct you on some techniques for avoiding falls.

The avoidance of falls and the encouragement of exercise have paradoxical elements. One might think that, to avoid falls, the most effective technique would be to sit all day. This would, of course, be a mistake because to do so would be to lose the clear benefits of muscle-pulling and weight-bearing exercise. Clearly, to move about is essential in maintaining your bones; thus, to move about safely is the objective.

Avoid heavy lifting. In fact, you would be well advised, in particular if you have already experienced a vertebral fracture, to avoid sudden bending. Activities that strain your skeleton, like jumping or twisting, or those in which you risk falling, should be avoided.

PLAY IT SAFE

Try and eliminate the obvious dangers around your home. The following safety checklist, based on recommendations from the National Osteoporosis Foundation and the American Medical Association, offers a good basic approach to inspecting your home for hazards:

- Floors. Remove all loose wires, cords, and throw rugs. Minimize clutter. Make sure rugs are anchored, especially on smooth, polished floors. Keep furniture in its accustomed place.
- Stairs. Make sure treads, rails, and rugs are secure. Are they properly lit? If your vision has dimmed, it may make sense to paint the walls on one or both sides of the stairway white to reflect the light overhead and make the stairs more visible. Banisters are important, too, on both interior and exterior steps.
- Bathrooms. Install grab bars and nonskid tape in the tub or shower. A handrail near the toilet may also be helpful.
- Lighting. Make sure halls, stairways, and entrances are well lit. Install night lights in your bathroom and bedroom. Turn lights on if you get up in the middle of the night.
- Kitchen. Install nonskid rubber mats near sink and stove. Clean spills immediately.
- Other Precautions. Wear sturdy, rubber-soled shoes and don't let your shoelaces trip you up. Keep your intake of alcoholic beverages to a minimum. Ask your doctor whether any of your medications might cause you to fall.

But the bottom line is that physical activity is an essential part of the osteoporosis patient's therapy. Inactivity, in fact, will only worsen your problem. So don't give up and retire to your rocking chair. Get up and go for a walk. It may not be comfortable, but chances are it will do you good—both physically and mentally.

After a Fractured Vertebra

If you have recently experienced a vertebral fracture, your pain may be sufficient that your desire to make virtually any movement is limited. Yet immobilization can serve to worsen your osteoporosis.

As a result, it is recommended in most cases to try to move

STRENGTHENING YOUR BACK

If osteoporosis has weakened your spine, you are unlikely to be able to restore a great deal of the lost bone mass. On the other hand, if you strengthen the muscles of the back, you may be able to minimize the discomforts and the risk of vertebral fractures.

Here is a sampling of the sort of muscle strengthening exercise you may find helpful. Be sure to discuss these and any exercises with your doctor or physical therapist before proceeding. All of these are done lying on your back.

LOWER BACK STRETCHES: Bending your legs at the knee, bring both legs to your chest. Hold them to your chest for a count of ten. Now do it one leg at a time: clench your left knee to your chest for a ten count, then your right for ten seconds. Gradually work up to ten repetitions of each of these bends.

TUMMY TIGHTENER: With your feet flat on the floor and knees bent, tighten your stomach and buttock muscles, thereby pressing your lower back to the floor. Hold for a count of ten, and repeat ten times.

LEG RAISES: With the left leg bent at the knee, lift your straightened right leg about six inches off the floor. Hold it there momentarily, then lower it slowly. Now do the same with your left leg. Repeat this pair of lifts ten times each.

HEAD AND SHOULDER LIFTS: With your knees bent, fold your arms across your chest. Now, keeping your neck stiff, lift your head and shoulders just off the floor. Hold for a count of five; repeat ten times.

about after a few days or a week have passed following the fracture. The pain will gradually lessen over a period of several weeks to a few months, so resume your activities gradually; use of a walker or cane may be well advised.

In most cases, you will be able to return to full activity over time, but take it at a reasonable pace. If you find that a period of exercise leaves your back very tired and weak, you may find that by taking periodic rests, lying down face up for an hour or so, will help you tolerate increasing amounts of movement.

Your doctor or a physical therapist may provide you with a regimen to follow. It may involve swimming, an excellent form of exercise that does not put undue strain on the skeleton.

Psychosomatic Aspects

More than a few books and magazines these days are investing thousands of words in the discussion of the relationship between the mind and the body. As the most responsible of those writings suggest, there is a correlation between stress and guilt and worry and some ailments. However, the fact is that for all osteoporosis patients, the problem is—and always has been—in their bodies and not in their heads.

Yet in dealing with osteoporosis, as with any chronic disease, one's attitude is critical. You must not rely on magical medications or your doctor's healing hands. They simply aren't enough. You must will yourself to fight the battle the best way you know how. But it won't be easy.

In our society, the unkempt or oddly attired man is often regarded as eccentric. But a woman of similar appearance? She is more likely to be thought unattractive. Fair or not, a woman's appearance is an important factor in determining how other people regard her.

To a woman with advanced osteoporosis, the characteristic loss of height, the bent posture of the dowager's hump, and the protruding abdomen are almost surely painful blows to her self-image. At the very least, finding flattering clothing is harder;

much worse, it may make her feel unattractive or old before her time. These feelings can only be exaggerated by the loss of mobility and independence that is often the result of hip fractures.

It is much easier to say than to do, but in dealing with a chronic condition the first step is to accept that it is there. You can't look at it as a terrible weight forever trying to pull you down; rather, your osteoporosis is just another of life's obstacles, a problem presented for your solution. In order to solve it, you must begin by making a deal with yourself, accepting the fact that your body is changing, perhaps seeming to age at a faster rate than those of your contemporaries.

In the next few pages, we'll talk about depression and anger, both of which are quite normal responses to the pain and deformity in one's life and body that osteoporosis brings. We'll also talk about stress and how life's pressures should be managed to help in the treatment of osteoporosis rather than to hinder it.

Depression and Anger

It is easy to understand why people with osteoporosis can become angry or depressed or both. After a painful fracture, whether the first or a later one, it may seem terribly unfair. You may feel angry at your fate and depressed at your condition.

These feelings are quite normal. In fact, depression often seems to occur in people who do not allow enough of their anger and frustration to surface. Don't deny the truth: you have osteoporosis and it has an effect on your life, so you must accept it.

Don't give up on living a normal, happy life. Adjustments may be necessary, of course, and some activities may have to be changed or eliminated, but you don't have to withdraw from things entirely.

Depression is a problem that has as many symptoms as it has sufferers, but among them are irritability; withdrawal; disturbed sleep; reduced or exaggerated eating; decreased concern with appearance; a sense that life has no value; persistent gloomy, negative thoughts; and slowed speech and body movements. If you find yourself feeling depressed or angry, you may wish to discuss matters with your doctor, especially if you are taking tranquilizers or if you consume a good deal of alcohol. Your doctor may recommend that you talk with a therapist trained in dealing with the psychological problems of chronic illness.

Stress

When an athlete works to get up for a game or a salesperson revs up for the next call, the "up" he or she is after is stress-induced. It is stress that allows us to adjust to the ordinary and extraordinary pressures of everyday life.

Stress is normal but, like most things, in excess it can be unhealthy. This is true for anyone, but it is even more so for the osteoporosis patient.

Think of excess stress as an illness, complete with symptoms, dangers, and treatments. The symptoms vary from one person to the next, but common ones are an overall feeling of tenseness, anxiety, or irritability; a general sense of fatigue; disturbed sleep; a reduced or exaggerated appetite; muscle tenseness; and difficulty in concentrating.

Stress may be the result of life's highs or lows. Marriage, the birth of a baby, the death of a friend or relative, retirement, the loss of a job or taking a new one are all stressful occurrences. Controlling stress and the impact it can have on your ability to control your life and your illness are important.

There are some simple strategies that may help. At times, they may be hard to follow, but try.

- Accept what you cannot change. No matter how willing you are to take on life's challenges, there is no point in doing battle with those forces you cannot change. Accept the facts, and use your energies to positive ends.
- Take life one day at a time. Try and focus on what is important today and not be distracted by the unknowns of next week

or a year from now. In the same way, negotiate your way around the obstacles before you, taking each as it comes.

- Try and do something each day you enjoy. Life's little pleasures can sometimes make the bigger problems seem less immense.
- Be reasonable in establishing goals and plans. Don't set goals that you can't possibly meet, as you'll only be disappointed when you fail and put pressure on yourself in the process.
- Incorporate a period of exercise into your daily schedule. Exercise and relaxation are a happy coupling.
- Use relaxation exercises at times of maximum stress. Your physical therapist may help you learn some appropriate ones.

Living with Pain

The first fact is the hardest to take: osteoporosis is chronic, meaning you will have to learn to live with it for the rest of life.

The second fact you already know: with osteoporosis, one of the key symptoms is pain. Though along with the other symptoms, the pain may come and go over time, you will have to live with it, too.

If you are one of those osteoporosis sufferers to whom the pain is not a constant concern, then you are lucky and unusual. For most people, dealing with osteoporosis involves learning how to manage the pain that accompanies the ailment.

Use the weapons your doctor has offered you in battling with pain, but don't expect the medication alone to make your discomfort go away. Follow his advice on exercise and rest, too, and obey his instructions.

Listen to what your body tells you: if it is complaining loudly and clearly that you are trying to do too much, stop. Pace yourself. Learn your limits, and don't exceed them. If you find that five hours of gardening puts you in bed for a week but three leaves you with no ill effects, put the observation to work. Doing less today may allow you to do something tomorrow instead of recovering from yesterday's exertions.

At the same time, don't allow the pain to control your life. You must control it. Learn to think about other things when the pain is uncomfortable. Keep active doing what you can. If your mind and body are occupied, you may find yourself too busy to hurt.

CHAPTER 3

Other Resources

Osteoporosis affects nearly twenty million Americans. In itself, that is a staggering and saddening statistic. However, the good news is that, because of the sheer number of sufferers, there is a growing pool of resources to help.

Not only is there a considerable bibliography (see Chapter 5) and an array of products (Chapter 4) available, but there are a diversity of healthcare professionals and associations to meet the needs of osteoporosis patients. It is these individuals and organizations that are the focus of this chapter.

This chapter is divided into two sections. The first concerns the professionals, the individuals who play specific roles in your healthcare, from the familiar family doctor to specialists like the orthopedic surgeon and the discharge planner. It is in this section that you will meet the guides who will help you negotiate the tricky medical landscape.

The second section introduces the organizations out there that also may be of help to you. Some of them, like those devoted to helping the disabled, will be of value to specific patients; others are more broad-based. Some associations offer group therapy, most have newsletters or other publications, many sponsor research. Virtually all can offer you some valuable services in getting the best care possible.

As a patient dealing with the course of a chronic illness like osteoporosis, you are forced to respond to sometimes unexpected events. In this chapter you will get a broad picture of the services out there to help you respond, and of the kinds of specific help available from medical professionals and concerned national and local organizations.

The Professionals

We live in a world where specialization rules. While the notion of a "family doctor" has made a notable comeback in recent years, the prevailing wisdom still argues strongly for expert consultation, especially when your complaint is unusual or serious.

If your osteoporosis is diagnosed early, your family doctor will probably be able to provide you with the medical advice and care you need (these days, by the way, the family doctor, perhaps a general practitioner or internist, is often termed the "primary care physician"). He or she should tell you about diet and exercise and about taking care to avoid certain physical stresses. However, if your osteoporosis is more advanced, or if you feel that you want special dietary or other consultation, your doctor may well refer you to a specialist.

Today there are many medical specialties which, as organized groups, set the rules for the training and certification of doctors. Among the specialists with whom you, as an osteoporosis patient, may work are the rheumatologist, the orthopedic surgeon and the physiatrist, or specialist in physical medicine.

Each has a different period of required training and different types of examinations; the requirements are, of course, tailored to the nature of the discipline and are meant to assure that those certified are competent. With pride in their discipline and with the desire to foster only the best possible performance, the various certifying bodies or boards often require years of practice under supervision and set very difficult examinations. In fact, "board certification" implies skills and knowledge that are well above the level required for state licensing as a physician.

Another modern trend has been toward more and more specialization, even in the face of public demand for more generalists and family doctors. However, many older physicians, despite having devoted much of their professional lives to certain fields of human illness, are not necessarily board certified; yet they may share or perhaps surpass the expertise of the younger, certified doctor. Thus, while it is important to be aware of your doctor's certificates and listings in specialty directories, such factors do not tell the whole story.

The Internist

An internist is a doctor trained in internal medicine who has gone on to become a specialist; the variety you are most likely to meet will be a rheumatologist, a specialist in bone and joint diseases including osteoporosis. He or she has not only an M.D. degree but has also completed additional training in rheumatology.

Becoming an internist involves spending a minimum of three years after medical school getting accredited training in the broad field of internal medicine. The three-year period is often divided into a year of internship and two of residency, but in any case the thirty-six months of training will have included at least twenty-four months of "meaningful patient responsibility." Two examinations must also be passed.

Having earned the right to be called an internist, the doctor who wishes to become a specialist in rheumatology must complete two additional years of full-time graduate training. There is another written examination to be passed, and the candidate must have his or her clinical competence attested to by the director of the rheumatology program. The result is a high level of expertise in the rheumatic diseases. The rheumatic diseases are sometimes thought of as solely those that affect the joints; but as the joints are between bones and are moved by muscles, perhaps thinking of the rheumatologist as one who specializes in musculoskeletal diseases is more appropriate. In any event, your rheumatologist will have a thorough knowledge of the complexities of bone formation and destruction as well as osteoporosis.

If you have any difficulty in finding a qualified rheumatologist, check with your county medical society or a local accredited hospital. The Osteoporosis Foundation or the Arthritis Foundation can help, as can other organizations discussed in the second half of this chapter.

Often a rheumatologist will work with a nurse who has received special training in rheumatology. In some cases, two or more rheumatologists will pool their resources to work together in a single office or clinic where x-ray resources, physical therapists, and other healthcare providers with special skills vis-à-vis osteoporosis are gathered.

Endocrinologist

Another type of internist, the endocrinologist, may be helpful to the osteoporosis patient. As we discussed in Chapters 1 and 2, many hormones are involved in the development and treatment of osteoporosis: estrogens, androgens, parathormone, and calcitonin are examples. The endocrinologist is an expert on the endocrine glands, the source of these hormones, and is an excellent adviser on sources, doses, and uses of hormones in therapy. A few endocrinologists actually work in an even narrower field, studying calcium, phosphorus, and bone metabolism, all as controlled by endocrine hormones. The patient with osteoporosis who finds a "bone and calcium" specialist will get excellent advice.

Nutritionist or Registered Dietitian

Because calcium and other nutrients are important in treating osteoporosis, you may need to consult a nutritionist or registered dietitian. Although both have essentially the same formal background—completion of a college curriculum in food, nutrition, or institutional management—the registered dietitian also has met the requirements of the American Dietetics Association and passed the national registration examination.

A nutritionist or registered dietitian can provide additional education to help you understand the principles and methods of a suitable diet to safeguard against bone loss. He or she can also counsel you in planning meals.

Orthopedic Surgeon

If you sustain a hip or wrist fracture, you will probably meet up with an orthopedic surgeon or orthopedist. Orthopedics is a surgical discipline concerned with the prevention or correction of disorders involving bones, joints, muscles, and supporting structures.

Like other medical specialists, the orthopedic surgeon is a doctor who has completed advanced training in his or her specialty. That means that in addition to medical school, he or she has completed a minimum of five years of postdoctoral education. Generally, this residency period will involve broad-based training in surgery, an orthopedic surgical residency in adult orthopedics, some time in children's orthopedics, and additional months dealing with fractures and traumas. Other requirements include passing a comprehensive examination.

In some circumstances, your orthopedist or rheumatologist may opt to use one or several nonsurgical methods, including physical manipulation, braces, or appliances. If surgery is judged not to be the proper course, you may find yourself in the hands of a physiatrist, physical therapist, or occupational therapist.

Physiatrist

In some cases your primary care physician may refer you to a physiatrist.

Physiatrists are medical doctors with a specialty in physical medicine. Physical medicine and rehabilitation, as the specialty is formally designated, is concerned with restoring useful function to damaged or injured joints or limbs through physical rather than surgical procedures. To become a physiatrist, four years of postgraduate residency training are required, of which three years must be in physical medicine and rehabilitation. The remaining year consists of experience in more general clinical skills in such areas as family practice, internal medicine, pediatrics, and general surgery. There are also written and oral examinations.

Generally, an orthopedic surgeon or rheumatologist knows enough about physical medicine to prescribe the exercises, special clothing, or equipment you need. However, a general practitioner or internist often will involve a physiatrist to establish an exercise program for deformity prevention and muscle maintenance.

Many physiatrists have special skills in pain-control treatments and local injections, but particularly in the wide range of exercises that can be helpful in maintaining or rebuilding function. Physiatrists sometimes direct the work of substantial departments or offices employing physical and occupational therapists.

Physical Therapist

If your osteoporosis is serious, you most likely will make the acquaintance of a physical therapist.

The physical therapist is not a medical doctor but is a licensed professional. Educational preparation differs (some physical therapists have bachelor's degrees, others have master's), but the curriculum includes coursework in anatomy, physiology, neuroanatomy, neurophysiology, and a variety of other areas. Some work independently in their own private offices. Others are employed within the offices of rheumatologists or orthopedic surgeons, while still others work in substantial programs supervised by physiatrists.

Generally the physical therapist treats osteoporosis or the results of other diseases or injuries by means of physical agents. These include heat, light, water, electronic or manual massage, and exercise.

The treatment is prescribed by your primary care physician or surgeon, often in cooperation with the physical therapist. The physical therapist (who is sometimes called a physiotherapist) is most likely to develop for you some combination of physiotherapy involving assisted and unassisted exercise to maintain range of motion and to build muscular strength. Some programs require the use of devices such as chairs, parallel bars, or other pieces of equipment that enable you to work on specific muscles. Your physical therapist may treat you in the hospital or at private offices. In some cases, he or she may even make house calls.

Occupational Therapist

The line between occupational and physical therapy varies from hospital to hospital. Like the physical therapist, the occupational therapist is not an M.D. but is a licensed professional who, under the guidance of a doctor, may introduce you to devices like canes, crutches, elevated toilet seats, shoes, and other products discussed in the last chapter.

Occupational therapists are skilled in evaluating the "livability" of a specific home or apartment for a handicapped person; improvements such as eliminating a doorway sill or putting in a bathroom wall bar can make a big difference.

The occupational therapist is also concerned with helping you in a broader sense. Vocational matters are considered: the goal is to reeducate you, to help you compensate for the loss of efficiency or ability that you may have incurred as a result of your osteoporosis. From both a sociological and a medical standpoint, the concern is to help you maintain or regain your self-sufficiency. According to the American Occupational Therapy Association (page 89):

Occupational therapy helps by working with the older adult to adapt to age-related changes such as decreased energy and vision; perform routine activities safely such as dressing and cooking; increase physical strength and endurance to maintain self-sufficiency; identify and use community resources such as transportation and household services; find community support groups such as senior centers and stroke clubs; cope with the normal losses of aging such as the death of a spouse or friend.

Other Healthcare Professionals

There are a multitude of other healthcare providers whom you may meet in your travels across the medical landscape. If you are hospitalized and require special services upon leaving, you are likely to make the acquaintance of a discharge planner. The discharge planner is responsible for coordinating the services you will require for the transition from hospital environment to home. This responsibility runs the gamut from filling out forms to arranging for equipment to other complex family, financial, and medical circumstances. Although the job designation of discharge planner is a relatively new one, social workers and nurses have long handled the responsibilities.

In cases where depression or other mental health concerns arise, a medical social worker may be called in. In cases where the problem is more severe, a psychologist or a psychiatrist may be consulted (the psychologist has a Ph.D., the psychiatrist is an M.D. with a specialty in psychiatry).

No doubt a pharmacist will fill your prescriptions for drugs; he or she can be an invaluable source of information regarding medications if there are things you don't understand.

Whether you meet only a few of these players or all of them, they, along with nurses and other personnel in the hospitals, clinics, and offices you may visit, constitute the team that is assembled to help treat your osteoporosis. They are there to help you: ask them questions and try to develop a relationship with them as you do with any expert to whom you look for guidance.

The Organizations

Make that call, write that letter, follow up on that lead. Drop a line to or telephone any of the following organizations if their concerns are yours. That is especially true if they are in your area.

You'll discover that these organizations offer a variety of services, from access to discussion groups or swimming therapy, to lectures and home food service, to home care and nursing help. Get in touch with them and find out.

Check your phone book, too, for local organizations. Ask your doctor and other patients for additional sources.

There are many other people like you out there, having to learn to deal with osteoporosis. You are not alone: get to know your peers, as they can best understand you, your problems, and your pain. And get all the help you can.

ACCENT
Gillum Road and High Drive
P.O. Box 700
Bloomington, Illinois 61702

Founded in the early 1950s by Raymond Cheever, this organization first began with the magazine *Accent On Living*. Cheever, recovering from polio, discovered that assistive devices were hard to find, so he set about providing "a means for disabled people to find out about products that were available but hard to find."

Today, *Accent On Living* magazine services its audience with information about vacations, products, projects, news of special interest to the disabled, and numerous uplifting stories of handicapped people who, despite their physical limitations, have become accomplished, happy, and successful. The magazine features many advertisements aimed specifically at the disabled. The magazine is published quarterly and costs $6.00 per year.

The Accent organization also has a computerized database that can access sources for thousands of products and publications in areas of special concern to the handicapped. Called Accent On Information, this service provides product and publication names and sources for a wide range of problems. The cost is $12.00 per search plus a photocopying cost of $.35 per page.

Accent also publishes a range of books and booklets (see page 142 for the *Accent On Living Buyer's Guide*).

AMERICAN ACADEMY OF ORTHOPAEDIC SURGEONS
222 South Prospect Avenue
Park Ridge, Illinois 60068-4085
(312) 823-7186

Founded in 1933, the American Academy of Orthopaedic Surgeons (AAOS) today is the largest medical association of musculoskeletal specialists, with more than 13,000 members worldwide. All members are board-certified orthopedic surgeons.

AAOS is concerned with continuing education for its membership, with monitoring legislative and governmental activities regarding orthopedics, and with public education. One of their publications concerns osteoporosis (page 135).

Contact AAOS for the names of surgeons in your area experienced in dealing with osteoporosis and other bone diseases.

AMERICAN ASSOCIATION OF RETIRED PERSONS
1909 K Street, NW
Washington, D.C. 20049
(202) 872-4700

AARP is a nonprofit, nonpartisan, social welfare, educational, and scientific membership organization. It is dedicated to helping older men and women achieve independence, dignity, and purpose. Active membership is open to all persons age fifty and older.

The organization produces health education programs available through thousands of local chapters. It also offers guaranteed enrollment in a number of group health insurance plans and maintains the AARP Pharmacy Service, which provides walk-in and mail-order services. Membership is $5.00 per year and includes a subscription to *Modern Maturity Magazine.*

AMERICAN DIETETIC ASSOCIATION
430 North Michigan Avenue
Chicago, Illinois 60610
(312) 751-6166

The American Dietetic Association is a membership group of nutritionists and dietitians. The association is concerned with dietary aspects of osteoporosis and can provide referral to local services and specialists in your area.

Write to the association for advice on proper nutrition and other materials suitable to osteoporosis prevention and treatment.

AMERICAN MEDICAL ASSOCIATION
535 North Dearborn Street
Chicago, Illinois 60610
(312) 751-6000

The largest membership organization of physicians, the AMA also serves as a source of information on specialists, facilities, and other matters relating to medicine. Write to the organization for information on osteoporosis or related medical matters, or if you need help in locating a physician or specialist in your area.

AMERICAN OCCUPATIONAL THERAPY ASSOCIATION, INC.
1383 Piccard Drive
P.O. Box 1725
Rockville, Maryland 20850-4375
(301) 948-9626

Founded in 1917, AOTA is the oldest allied health professional society. Along with the AMA, it accredits occupational therapy programs, certifies occupational therapists, and supports research efforts in therapeutic theories and techniques. It also runs continuing education programs and publishes a variety of periodicals for professionals as well as for the lay public (see "Daily Activities After Your Hip Surgery, page 147).

Your doctor or hospital is likely to refer you to an occupational therapist if one is required in treating your osteoporosis. However, if you have trouble finding a qualified occupational therapist nearby, write or call the association for a referral to a therapist or rehabilitation facility in your area.

AMERICAN PHARMACEUTICAL ASSOCIATION
2215 Constitution Avenue, NW
Washington, D.C. 20027
(202) 628-4410

The association produces and distributes materials on a variety of drugs and related subjects. Write to them for information on brand name and generic drugs, over-the-counter preparations, drug interactions, child safety, or other matters related to the use and abuse of medicines.

AMERICAN PHYSICAL THERAPY ASSOCIATION
1111 North Fairfax Street
Alexandria, Virginia 22314
(703) 684-APTA

APTA is, as its name suggests, a professional association for physical therapists. If you are having difficulty in finding a qualified physical therapist in your area, write or call the association for the address of the chapter nearest you which, in turn, can provide referrals to therapists and facilities in your area and any other available patient and community services.

THE ARTHRITIS FOUNDATION
1314 Spring Street
Atlanta, Georgia 30309
(800) 282-7023

Perhaps the key source of patient information on arthritis in the United States, the Arthritis Foundation is a nonprofit organization with branch chapters in virtually every state.

Founded in 1948, the foundation is a national, voluntary health organization whose programs include support for scientific research, the training of specialists, and community assistance programs for arthritis patients. These community programs vary from chapter to chapter, but support groups, arthritis clinics, home care programs, exercise classes, and rehabilitation services are among those offered.

The foundation is concerned with raising funds to forward its research and service goals and is active in government affairs insofar as people with osteoporosis are affected.

If you have arthritis, osteoporosis, or both, consult the chapter nearest you. The chapters provide a variety of useful publications at no charge, as well as guidance regarding specialists, clinics, and other local agencies that may be of help to you in dealing with the economic, emotional, physical, and medical problems attendant to arthritis and osteoporosis. The organization publishes a magazine, *Arthritis Today,* six times yearly. Membership and a subscription cost $15.00 per year.

An associated organization is the Arthritis Health Professions Association. It is made up of physical and occupational therapists, nurses, psychologists, social workers, and other healthcare professionals concerned with arthritis patients.

A related group is the American Juvenile Arthritis Organization.

CLEARINGHOUSE ON THE HANDICAPPED
U.S. Department of Education
Switzer Building
Room 3132
Washington, D.C. 20202

Established under the auspices of the Rehabilitation Act of 1973, the agency's objectives are to provide information and data on services and programs for the handicapped, as well as research and recent medical and scientific developments.

The Clearinghouse on the Handicapped provides statistical and other resource information to organizations and issues publications for the general public. Its scope includes vocational training, employment, and educational concerns for a wide range of handicapped people.

GOODWILL INDUSTRIES OF AMERICA, INC.
9200 Wisconsin Avenue
Bethesda, Maryland 20814
(301) 530-6500

Goodwill Industries is a familiar fixture in many communities as a place where used clothing and household goods are contributed for repair and eventual resale through Goodwill thrift shops. However, this activity is a means to an end.

In fact, local Goodwill Industries provide important services to the disabled: they offer vocational evaluation, training, employment, and job placement services. If you are disabled, feel able to seek employment, but have no apparent options before you, check with your local Goodwill Industries or with the national offices.

HANDICAPPED ORGANIZED WOMEN, INC.
P.O. Box 35481
Charlotte, North Carolina 28235
(704) 376-4735

Handicapped Organized Women is a nonprofit organization founded "to provide emotional support by enabling every woman to reach her fullest potential; to aid in the education of disabled women and the community by developing a positive image; to be as independent as can be, as dependent as need be, and to understand the difference; to foster growth and unity through the sharing of experiences."

Founded in 1979, HOW now has 145 chapters in forty-three states. The brainchild of Deborah McKeithan (who continues as its president), HOW "was started because I needed it and it wasn't there." McKeithan, who has multiple sclerosis and epilepsy, has had a stroke, and is legally blind, founded the national organization with a grant from the W. Clement and Jessie V. Stone Foundation.

HOW publishes a newsletter, *The National News,* which offers information about the organization, other sources of information, and reviews of new publications. HOW lobbies actively on healthcare and other issues of concern to the handicapped. Its local chapters are involved with volunteer work with disabled people and the development of employment programs to help the disabled to work. If you have severe osteoporosis and suffer a resultant disability, you may contact the local chapter of HOW through the national headquarters.

MELPOMENE INSTITUTE FOR WOMEN'S HEALTH
    RESEARCH
2125 East Hennepin Avenue
Minneapolis, Minnesota 55413
(612) 378-0545

The Melpomene Institute for Women's Health Research is "dedicated to discovering, through well-founded scientific inquiry, the facts inherent in physical activity for women. By learning how exercise specifically benefits women, as well as what problems it may cause, Melpomene provides practical information to women seeking to make informed choices about their lifestyles.''

The nonprofit organization, which is named for the first woman Olympic marathoner, conducts ongoing studies on the relationship between physical activity and osteoporosis, between exercise and pregnancy, and on athletic amenorrhea, or the cessation of menstruation due to exercise. A membership organization supported by grants as well as fees, the Melpomene Institute conducts conferences, publishes *The Melpomene Report* (three times a year), and maintains a resource center. It also makes available an information packet on osteoporosis which contains a wide variety of articles on calcium, estrogen, and exercise. The cost is $5.50.

If you would like further information, write or call the institute. Younger, active women might well benefit from joining or from reviewing other information packages available from Melpomene on such subjects as exercise and pregnancy and athletic amenorrhea.

NATIONAL ARTHRITIS AND MUSCULOSKELETAL AND SKIN DISEASES CLEARINGHOUSE
National Institutes of Health
U.S. Public Health Service
Department of Health and Human Services
Box AMS
Bethesda, Maryland 20892
(301) 468-3235

Established in 1978, the clearinghouse operates under the auspices of the National Institute of Arthritis and Musculoskeletal and Skin Diseases (NIAMS, see page 94), which is, in turn, part of the National Institutes of Health funded by the federal government.

The NIAMS Clearinghouse identifies itself as ''a national

resource designed to help health professionals identify educational materials and programs." Because of limited resources, the clearinghouse cannot service the needs of the lay public. Rather, its concern is to provide information to health educators, physicians, nurses, pharmacists, health planners and policy analysts, and other health professionals.

One notable service the clearinghouse offers is access to a computerized bibliographic database of health information. Called Combined Health Information Database (CHID), it can save your physician or other members of your healthcare team valuable time otherwise lost in searching through libraries, as CHID "provides abstracts and bibliographic citations to articles in major health journals, books, reports, pamphlets, hard-to-find information sources, and health education programs." The database contains more than 30,000 citations and is updated quarterly. For more information about CHID, contact the Division of Health Education, Center for Health Promotion and Education, Centers for Disease Control, Atlanta, Georgia 30333. Telephone: (404) 329-3492.

The clearinghouse also publishes bibliographies, directories, and reference sheets for physicians and other health professionals. It distributes information to the health professionals on its mailing list, for whom its services are free of charge. Your doctor can contact the clearinghouse with specific questions.

THE NATIONAL INSTITUTE OF ARTHRITIS AND MUSCULOSKELETAL AND SKIN DISEASES
Building 31
Room 9A04
National Institutes of Health
Bethesda, Maryland 20205

The National Institute of Arthritis and Musculoskeletal and Skin Diseases (NIAMS) is a research institution. Funded by the federal government, NIAMS is charged with leading and coordinating the federal government's biomedical research efforts into musculoskeletal disorders, including osteoporosis. It was created in 1986 as a separate institute (formerly, musculoskeletal disease research was conducted under the auspices of the National Institute of Arthritis, Diabetes, and Digestive and Kidney Diseases).

The institute provides support for a coordinated program of basic and clinical research and research training concerning the causes, prevention, diagnosis, and treatment of a large number of diverse diseases, including osteoporosis, osteogenesis imperfecta, and Paget's disease. NIAMS also conducts and supports information and education activities for the public through the Office and Health Research Reports and the National Arthritis and Musculoskeletal and Skin Disease Information Clearinghouse (see page 93), which collects and disseminates materials on these diseases primarily to health professionals.

The work of NIAMS is conducted in intramural and extramural programs, the former by government scientists on the campus of the National Institutes of Health and the latter primarily by university scientists in their hospitals and clinics across the United States. The intramural program includes scientists working in laboratories on fundamental aspects of bones, muscles, and so on, as well as physicians conducting clinical studies in the Warren Grant Magnuson Clinical Center, the research hospital of the National Institutes of Health near Washington, D.C.

The much larger extramural program of NIAMS is a research support program making grants to groups of scientific investigators mostly in the United States, though some grant recipients work overseas. The scientists and doctors decide on the investigational path they think most important and ask NIAMS for the money to travel that path.

NATIONAL OSTEOPOROSIS FOUNDATION
1625 Eye Street, NW
Suite 1011
Washington, D.C. 20006
(202) 223-2226

Founded in 1984, NOF exists to focus national attention on osteoporosis. It is the only national voluntary health agency whose aim is to reduce the prevalence of osteoporosis.

NOF is proceeding on several fronts. Through public information efforts involving posters, press releases, the establishment of a National Osteoporosis Prevention Week, and media activity in magazines and on television, it is trying to alert the general public to prevention techniques. The foundation is also concerned with educating physicians through its publishing activity and by organizing conferences and symposia. It offers research grants for scientists and is starting to organize local chapters across the country to provide more direct assistance in specific localities.

The foundation is also a membership organization; annual dues are $20.00 for the layperson ($10.00 for those aged sixty-five and older). Membership entitles you to a subscription to the quarterly newsletter, *The Osteoporosis Report;* a free copy of the handout "Osteoporosis: A Woman's Guide"; discounts on other publications; and information about local chapters and patient support groups. The cost of joining is tax-deductible. Professional and physician memberships are more expensive but offer discounts on publications and reduced registration fees for conferences, workshops, and symposia.

NATIONAL REHABILITATION INFORMATION CENTER
4407 Eighth Street, NE
Washington, D.C. 20017
(800) 34-NARIC

NARIC is an information source: it maintains two databases concerned with disability-related research, support services, and consumer products. These resources include information on topics as varied as disability and the family and sexuality, guides to resources in individual states, and a miscellany of products and services to help people with disabilities.

The ABLEDATA database is an index of more than 14,000 commercially available products. From fishing rods to power tools, ABLEDATA contains a wealth of products helpful for personal care, home management, mobility, communication, and recreation. Each product reference contains the name, availability, description, cost, manufacturer, and, in many cases, commentary or evaluation of the product.

The REHABDATA database indexes more than 16,000 articles on issues related to the disabled.

NARIC encourages not only researchers and counselors but the disabled, their families, teachers, and medical professionals to take advantage of their capabilities. The fee for searches is usually nominal; call the 800-number for further information.

CHAPTER 4

Self-Help

Every case of osteoporosis is unique, yet all patients share one major concern: upon learning you have it, you inevitably begin to worry that the ailment will increasingly limit daily activities.

As we saw in Chapter 2, there are a variety of treatments that your doctor, with your cooperation, can select from in order to develop an appropriate plan of care for your individual case. In somewhat the same way, this chapter will introduce you to a number of strategies that may help you go about your daily life as normally as possible.

To begin with, you will learn about nutrition: what you eat can, in many cases, have a significant impact on your osteoporosis. We will also talk about exercise because, once again, physical activity can help you in your fight. Finally, the concluding section of this chapter will address a considerable array of products and offer buying advice for everyday and specialty items of special significance to the osteoporosis sufferer.

Nutritional Therapies

As you now know, calcium, vitamin D, and other nutrients all have roles in treating and preventing many cases of osteoporosis. But before discussing strategies for emphasizing those nutrients in your diet, let's take a "big picture" approach.

The simple fact is that a proper, balanced diet makes anyone "healthier" in a general sense. Whether you have osteoporosis or not, you will be healthier (and probably happier, too) if you eat a sensible, varied diet that contains all the nutrients your body needs.

There are a multitude of rules and advisories to follow in eating a balanced diet. One of the easiest sets of guidelines is to eat, on a daily basis, the following foods:

- 2 servings of protein (meat, fish, poultry, beans, eggs)
- 4 to 6 servings of fruit or vegetables (at least one green leafy vegetable and one citrus fruit)
- 4 to 6 servings of breads and cereals
- 2 servings of milk and dairy products
- 6 to 8 glasses of fluids

Try and consume a diet consistent with this simple plan as you incorporate foods high in calcium.

Getting Your Calcium

The best sources of calcium are milk and other dairy products and, in fact, Americans normally get 80 percent of their calcium from dairy products. You should drink at least one glass of milk a day. Four will give you 1,000 milligrams (1 gram) of calcium, which fulfills the Recommended Dietary Requirements for premenopausal women. Keep in mind, however, that lowfat or skim milk is preferable to minimize calories and cholesterol intake.

Fish that can be eaten with their bones, like canned salmon and sardines, are also excellent dietary sources of calcium. Leafy green vegetables contain substantial amounts of calcium, especially cabbage and collard greens. Not far behind are kale and mustard and turnip greens.

However, the amount of calcium that your body can absorb and utilize from green vegetables appears to be lower than that from dairy products. One reason is that green vegetables also contain phytic acid; this will bind to the calcium, reducing the body's ability to absorb it.

Soybeans (and tofu, a curd made from soybeans) are a good source of calcium. Other beans are rich in calcium, too, including navy, pinto, and chickpeas. Almonds and brazil nuts are also good sources of calcium. Lower on the list but nonetheless rich in calcium are walnuts, cashews, peanuts, lentils, peas, and a

CALCIUM-RICH FOODS

The following foods are rich in calcium:

Food	Serving Size	Calcium (mg)
Beans, dried, cooked	1 cup	90
Buttermilk	1 cup	285
Cheese, blue	1 ounce	150
Cheese, cheddar	1 ounce	191
Cheese, colby	1 ounce	194
Cheese, muenster	1 ounce	203
Cheese, Swiss	1 ounce	272
Collard, fresh	1/2 cup	179
Collard, frozen	1/2 cup	149
Kale, fresh	1/2 cup	103
Kale, frozen	1/2 cup	79
Milk, 2% lowfat	1 cup	297
Milk, skim	1 cup	302
Milk, whole	1 cup	291
Molasses, blackstrap	1 tablespoon	137
Oysters, raw	1 cup	226
Salmon (canned, with bones)	3 ounces	167
Sardines (with bones)	3 ounces	372
Shrimp, canned	3 ounces	99
Turnip greens, fresh	1/2 cup	126
Turnip greens, frozen	1/2 cup	98
Yogurt, lowfat plain	1 cup	415
Yogurt, with fruit	1 cup	389

variety of other foods including whole wheat cereals, brown rice, broccoli, chard, potatoes, okra, and lentils. (For easy reference, see the table of calcium-rich foods, above.)

In short, a daily menu that includes individual portions of two calcium-rich foods like almonds, broccoli, canned fish (with bones), kelp, tofu, tortillas, kale, turnips, or collard greens, macaroni and cheese, pizza, beef tacos, and cheese or meat enchiladas, will supply more than 400 milligrams of calcium. Along with milk or calcium supplements (see page 60) you should be able to fulfill the Recommended Dietary Allowance.

LACTOSE INTOLERANCE: Lactose is the principal carbohydrate found in milk. As babies, we have an enzyme in our digestive system, called lactase, that allows us to digest the lactose.

Lactase usually is present and active all our lives, but in some people its activity diminishes early. In those who develop what is known as "lactose intolerance," the most common pattern is that by eight or nine years of age, a child is no longer able to digest lactose efficiently.

The result is that the lactose arrives in the intestines undigested, where it is broken down by bacteria. The result is gas, bloating, and abdominal pain. Lactic acid is also produced, which irritates the intestine and causes diarrhea. Thus, characteristic symptoms of lactose intolerance vary from minor abdominal discomfort to bloating, flatulence, abdominal pain, and even explosive diarrhea only minutes after eating lactose-rich foods.

Only Europeans, particularly western Europeans and their descendants, maintain high levels of lactase into adult life. In fact, by the age of six, one's lactose activity is reduced to a tenth of the level during infancy in roughly 70 percent of the world's people.

Most who are lactose intolerant can consume some milk or milk products. Up to one cup of milk at a sitting is commonly found to be digestible without unpleasant symptoms. As a result, eliminating all foods rich in lactose is not generally necessary. Many people also find that drinking milk with solid foods helps its digestion. When milk is taken in with solid food, the rate at which the milk is presented to the intestine for absorption is reduced, giving the limited supply of lactase a better chance of digesting it.

Whole and chocolate milk contain fat, which slows down the rate at which the digestive system works, so it is better absorbed than skim milk. Yogurt is better tolerated because it contains some lactase, though that advantage is lost when yogurt is pasteurized.

If none of these strategies work for you, you might try lactase-hydrolyzed milk. It is made by incubating milk or other milk products with lactase for twenty-four hours. This reduces the lactose content by 40 to 90 percent, thereby lessening the symptoms of lactose intolerance.

COOKING FOR CALCIUM

SOUP IT UP: Here's a trick for cooks who make their own soups or stocks: When you use bones in making stock, add a little vinegar. The vinegar will help dissolve the calcium in the bones, making the resultant stock richer in calcium. Boiling the stock prior to adding the vegetables will dissipate the vinegar smell.

TRY OUT TOFU: It's like cheese, only it's made from soybeans. It's low in fat and calories but rich in calcium. It can be eaten plain, or served with all kinds of soups, salads, egg dishes, or even desserts. It takes on the flavors of the foods it is prepared with. Find it fresh in the produce section of your grocery store.

BAKING BREAD: Add powered milk to your dough to increase its calcium content.

USE THE YOGURT: It can be used in dips and salad dressings, even as a dessert topping, and it's eminently snackable.

The Other Dietary Factors

There are reasons to believe that other nutrients and food substances may have an effect on the development of osteoporosis. The evidence varies from very solid (we are quite sure of the importance of vitamin D) to rather conjectural (is it really protein or some other unidentified factor that, when consumed in large amounts, leads to a net loss of body calcium?). In any case, there is evidence that each of the following nutrients has an impact on your calcium status, and it makes good sense to take sensible precautions regarding each of them.

VITAMIN D: Vitamin D is on the recommended list for reasons discussed in detail earlier: in short, your body needs it to absorb calcium.

Because vitamin D is formed in the skin upon exposure to sunlight, you probably have sufficient amounts of the vitamin available to fulfill your body's needs if you spend a reasonable amount of time out of doors on a daily basis. However, if you are bedridden or tend to keep your skin largely covered when outside, you should pay attention to the amount of vitamin D-rich foods you consume.

The Recommended Dietary Allowance is 400 international units daily; so if you must rely on your diet as your sole source of the vitamin, you'll find yourself drinking lots of milk and eating much fatty fish and eggs. Another option is taking a multivitamin supplement, but check to make sure it contains the requisite amount of vitamin D.

VITAMIN A: For all the benefits offered by vitamin A, you should be aware that megadoses (over 4,000 international units) of vitamin A have been shown by the American Society for Bone and Mineral Research to lead to bone loss. Avoid taking large quantities of vitamin A.

PHOSPHORUS: Another nutrient that has a major impact upon your body's use of calcium is phosphorus. As we discussed in Chapter 1, your bones contain substantial amounts of this essential mineral.

We also know that your body's ability to absorb calcium is affected by the presence of phosphorus: the more phosphorus you consume, the less calcium your body will get. Thus, in planning your diet, especially if you are in the midst of or have passed through menopause, you should beware an imbalance in your calcium/phosphorus intake.

In practice, this means that a diet designed to lower your risk for osteoporosis should not only be high in calcium but should also be low in phosphorus.

The major sources of phosphorus in the diet are red meats and carbonated soft drinks. Some foods have an extraordinarily high phosphorus-to-calcium ratio: foods such as beef liver, bologna, fried chicken, corn on the cob, frankfurters, ground beef, ham, lamp chops, and pork chops have ratios between 15 to 1 and 45 to 1, which is very bad for calcium absorption. In contrast, many green leafy vegetables (like spinach and lettuce) have more calcium than phosphorus; therefore, calcium absorption is likely to be greater. Many carbonated soft drinks that contain phosphoric acid contain no calcium at all. On the other hand, dairy products contain approximately equal amounts of calcium and phosphorus.

The overall content of calcium and phosphorus in the diet is important, but so is the time at which these two nutrients are consumed in relation to one another. The more time that elapses between the ingestion of two minerals, the better, lest they combine in the intestinal tract to form an unabsorbable compound.

Meals that emphasize calcium-rich foods are better for you if they do not contain phosphorus-rich foods. Thus, calcium from the sour cream in the baked-potato-and-steak meal is not absorbed as well as from the late-evening-ice-cream snack. A good idea is to emphasize calcium in snack foods.

Consult the table of foods rich in phosphorus (see page 106). Adjust your selection of foods and dietary practice appropriately.

SALT: As a general rule, the more salt you consume, the more salt you excrete. Unfortunately, that also means that you will excrete more calcium as well. Salt contains sodium, and the high sodium intake forces the kidneys to excrete more sodium. Along with the excess sodium, the kidneys will also pass calcium out of your body.

It is not necessary to go on a low-sodium diet to protect your bones from osteoporosis, but if you are a "salt-oholic" you should reduce your consumption of salt, and not only for the health of your bones. Start with some mild restrictions on your sodium intake.

Begin by reducing the amount of table salt you use. Add none at table, and use no more than one teaspoon during cooking. You should also avoid pickled foods and extremely salty foods.

VITAMIN C: Vitamin C performs a number of important tasks, including aiding in iron absorption and in keeping the teeth and gums healthy. One of its lesser but nevertheless important contributions is in helping in calcium absorption. As a result, it makes sense to plan your diet so that you eat foods rich in vitamin C,

PHOSPHORUS-RICH FOODS

The following foods are rich in phosphorus:

Food	Serving Size	Phosphorus (mg)
Almonds	1 ounce	126
Apricots, dried	3 ounces	102
Brains, cooked	4 ounces	389
Bran	1 ounce	257
Brazil nuts	1 ounce	169
Cereal, whole grain	1 ounce	97
Cheese	2 ounces	163–432
Chocolate, milk	3 ounces	119–206
Cocoa	1 gram	189
Fish, cooked	4 ounces	143–572
Kidneys, cooked	4 ounces	411
Liver, cooked	4 ounces	212
Milk	1 cup	226
Peanuts	1 ounce	107
Peas, cooked	1 cup	86
Walnuts	1 ounce	146

such as citrus fruits, berries, and cantaloupe, at the same time as you consume calcium-rich foods.

OXALATES AND PHYTATES: Oxalate is a food substance found in green vegetables, including asparagus, beet greens, dandelion greens, rhubarb, sorrel, and spinach. Phytates are compounds containing phosphorus found in the husks of certain grains, in particular bran and oatmeal. During digestion, oxalates and phytates combine with calcium, resulting in insoluble compounds that your body cannot absorb.

These foods needn't be eliminated from your diet, but when planning your meals you should avoid scheduling the intake of oxalate- and phytate-rich foods at the times you consume foods rich in calcium. Also avoid taking calcium supplements at the same time as you eat food rich in these substances (see tables of foods containing phytates and oxalates, opposite).

PHYTATE-CONTAINING FOODS

The following foods are high in phytate:

Food	Serving Size	Phytate (mg)
Almonds	1 ounce	366
Apple, raw	1 medium	94
Beans, green, raw	2 ounces	377
Beans, lima, raw	2 ounces	509
Brazil nuts	1 ounce	514
Bread, rye	1 slice	235
Bread, whole wheat	1 slice	163
Cereal, All-Bran	1 ounce	679
Cereal, granola	1 ounce	175
Cereal, Shredded Wheat	1 ounce	415
Cocoa, dry	1 tablespoon	94
Lentils, raw	2 ounces	248
Oatmeal, cooked	1/2 cup	133
Peanuts	1 ounce	214
Popcorn, popped	1 cup	37
Sesame seeds	1 ounce	1,319
Walnuts	1 ounce	217
Wheat germ	1 tablespoon	244

OXALATE-RICH FOODS

The following foods are high in oxalates:

Beans, baked in tomato sauce
Beans, green, wax or dried
Beets
Blueberries or blackberries
Celery
Chocolate
Cocoa
Collard greens
Dandelion greens
Eggplant
Grapes
Kale
Lemon peel
Mustard greens
Okra
Parsley
Peppers, green
Raspberries
Soybean curd
Spinach
Squash, summer
Strawberries
Tangerines
Tea
Watercress
Wheat germ

FIBER: The best source of dietary fiber (or roughage, as it was once more commonly called) are grains, though many fruits and vegetables also are rich in fiber. Fiber promotes good digestion: it is indigestible, passes directly through the digestive tract unchanged, and provides bulk for the stool. However, just as the ingestion of fiber helps avoid constipation and other intestinal problems by speeding waste matter out of the body, its very efficiency leads to the elimination of much calcium as well.

Calcium and fiber bind naturally, so as with phytates and oxalates you should avoid eating fiber-rich foods when eating foods high in calcium or with calcium supplements.

DIETARY FIBER-RICH FOODS

The following foods are high in dietary fiber:

Food	Serving Size	Fiber (g)
Almonds	1/2 cup	7
Beans, baked	1/2 cup	7.3
Beans, green	1/2 cup	2.8
Bran	1/2 cup	15.4
Bread, rye	1 slice	.13
Bread, whole wheat	1 slice	.4
Broccoli, cooked	1 cup	4.1
Brussels sprouts, cooked	1 cup	2.9
Cabbage, cooked	3/4 cup	2.1
Carrots, cooked	3/4 cup	3.7
Cereal, All-Bran	1 cup	19
Cereal, Grape-Nuts	1/2 cup	4.7
Cereal, Shredded Wheat	1 biscuit	3
Corn, cooked	1 ear	6.6
Corn, canned	1/2 cup	7.3
Cornflakes	1 cup	2.8
Lettuce, raw	1 cup	.75
Oatmeal	1/2 cup	8.4
Peanuts, roasted	1/2 cup	5.8
Potatoes, baked	1	3
Prunes, with pits	5 large	8.0
Raisins	1/2 ounce	1
Spinach	1/2 cup	3
Walnuts	1/2 cup	3.1

PROTEIN: Protein has been demonstrated to increase calcium absorption. However, it also has been shown to increase calcium excretion. The main source of dietary protein is meat. Since most of us consume generous, if not excessive, amounts of meat, we also are losing substantial amounts of calcium.

Once again, this does not argue for the elimination of meat from the diet, but moderation. One approach would be to limit meat to one meal a day and reduce portion sizes. Keep in mind that dairy products being used to supply dietary calcium also contain significant amounts of protein; hence, there is no need to worry about protein deficiency.

Vegetarians, particularly ovo-lacto vegetarians (those who consume eggs and dairy products but no meat), have a lower incidence of osteoporosis than meat eaters. This is probably because of the lower protein and phosphorus content of their diets. A well-balanced vegetarian diet which allows milk and milk products is probably the best diet for the prevention of osteoporosis. The closer we all come to eating such a diet, the better, as the more restrictive vegetarian-type diets tend to be too low in calcium to supply the body's needs.

OTHER CONCERNS: Try and limit (or eliminate) your consumption of coffee, which interferes with your body's ability to absorb calcium. Limit alcohol, too.

Worried About Weight?

If you're concerned that consuming lots of dairy products will cause you to put on those pounds you've long fought to keep off, don't be. Although it's true that dairy products are higher in calories than many foods, there are strategies you can employ to minimize the risk of weight gain.

For instance, drink skim milk rather than whole milk; eat yogurt rather than ice cream. Cottage cheese, though high in phosphorus, is also a good choice for weight watchers.

More importantly, get your exercise. Ample exercise, as we will discuss in the next section, is essential to developing bone mass and is equally important to maintaining firm control of your weight.

Exercise Programs

Exercise, along with an adequate supply of calcium, is your best defense against the debilitating effects of osteoporosis.

The notion that exercise has an effect on bone development is hardly new. As early as 1892, a German researcher suggested that the mechanical forces of movement caused changes in bone. Although researchers are still debating the issue, a number of findings do suggest the significance of physical activity.

The studies vary. Scandinavian studies have found that ballet dancers have denser bones in their lower extremities and that tennis players have more bone mass in their dominant arms. Studies of baseball pitchers and cross-country runners have produced similar results. On the basis of such studies, researchers have concluded that bones respond specifically to environmental stresses put upon them.

While the amount of exercise attempted by a patient with a long history of fractures is likely to be less than that appropriate for one who is years away from such dangers, the point is the same: regular, reasonable exercise is a crucial part of the fight against osteoporosis.

The purpose of physical activity for you, the osteoporosis patient, is twofold. One, you will be attempting to restore lost bone mass or at least to prevent further losses. Two, you will be trying to improve your musculature in order to help prevent future falls, fractures, and deformities.

If you are working to prevent osteoporosis, your goal is simpler: you want to develop maximum bone mass so that the gradual, inevitable erosion of bones in later years will not leave your skeleton dangerously weakened.

Not all exercises are created equal. No doubt you've already read and heard more than you ever wanted to know about aerobic exercise (the variety in which sustained activity provides benefit to the heart and lungs as well as the muscles) versus anaerobic exercise (in which activity is limited to short bursts of vigorous exercise). To put it another way: running provides nonstop (and therefore aerobic) exercise, benefiting your heart and lungs; miscellaneous sit-ups and push-ups (anaerobic exercise) benefit your muscles but do not challenge your heart and lungs.

The fact is you need to get weight-bearing exercise, as we discussed in Chapter 2 (page 38), but the question of how much exercise is needed for skeletal fitness is still being studied. In general, however, good aerobic fitness and skeletal fitness both result from sound exercise programs. Until researchers can quantify what exactly is appropriate for skeletal fitness, it is advisable to work out with the goals of aerobic exercise in mind. If you can follow these established ground rules for cardiovascular fitness, it is likely that your skeleton will get the exercise it needs to avoid bone loss and to add mass.

As preventive exercise, jogging, walking, tennis, bicycling, dancing, cross-country skiing, rope jumping, and other activities that combine movement with stress on the limbs are recommended. Weight-training with free weights or on Nautilus, Universal, or other machines can also be valuable. Slightly riskier forms of exercise are gymnastics, basketball, and volleyball.

However, if you have osteoporosis, certain of these activities are best avoided. Jogging, for example, subjects the skeleton to a constant pounding: every stride concludes with the entire body weight shifting onto the lead foot, stressing the spine and hip along the way. For the healthy thirty-year-old, jogging might help develop bone mass; for the osteoporosis patient, it could increase the risk of fracture. If you already have osteoporosis, avoid jogging and, again, be sure to discuss any exercise program with your doctor. Your doctor may recommend a specific program, but appropriate exercise for the older woman includes walking, riding a stationary bicycle, and working out on a rowing machine.

Note, however, that although swimming may be the prescribed exercise for the osteoporosis patient recovering from a vertebral fracture, it is thought by many physicians to be a poor exercise for lowering the risk of osteoporosis in the younger, healthier

EXERCISE IMPERATIVES

DO IT REGULARLY: Establish a schedule for your exercise. You'll need to work out a minimum of three times a week for twenty minutes or more.

DETERMINE YOUR TARGET ZONE: In order to get maximum benefit, you need to get your heart pumping more than normal, to get the blood coursing through your arteries and feeding your muscles the extra oxygen they'll need. One method of measuring whether you are getting enough exercise for physical conditioning is by simply taking your pulse.

Periodically count the number of heartbeats per minute (your pulse rate) as you work out and determine an average. Then compare that number to what is called your "target zone." The target zone is calculated by subtracting your age from 220, and then determining 70 percent and 85 percent of that number. If you are forty years old, for example, multiply 180 (220 − 40) by .70 and .85. Your target zone, then, is between 126 and 153. That means that during vigorous exercise, your pulse rate should fall between those numbers for full cardiac benefit. If your heart is beating faster, you're working too hard; if it's beating slower, you're not getting maximum cardiac benefit.

LOOSEN UP: Make sure that you allow at least five minutes before and after each workout to loosen your muscles and to allow your heart and lungs to grow accustomed to the extra activity you are demanding of them.

CHECK WITH YOUR DOCTOR: If you live a sedentary life, are over thirty-five, or suffer from any chronic disease, an exercise-tolerance test is recommended before starting any exercise program. This should also be done if you experience chest pain, irregular heartbeat, or shortness of breath; have high blood pressure or an elevated cholesterol count; are a smoker; are overweight; or have a relative who had a heart attack before the age of fifty.

person. This is because the water, rather than the bones, supports the weight of the body, so it is not a weight-bearing exercise. Although at least one recent study contradicts this belief, until further investigations are completed, it seems sensible to find a weight-bearing variety of exercise. If none works for you, swimming is certainly far better than inactivity.

If you are not in good physical condition, you must start exercising sensibly. It only makes sense to begin a physical fitness program at a gradual pace: remember, you aren't running a race. The idea is to establish an exercise habit that you can live with for years.

The following chart may be useful for establishing a walking regimen:

WEEK OF PROGRAM	DISTANCE (Miles)	TIME (Minutes/Mile)
1–2	1	20
2–3	1	17–20
4–6	1	15
7–8	1.5	15
9–10	1.5	14

If you stop exercising for more than two weeks, start up at a lower level and build up again in the usual way.

On the other hand, if you feel you are already in relatively good physical condition, you may want to start a little faster. A walking regimen for you might be as follows:

WEEK OF PROGRAM	DISTANCE (Miles)	TIME (Minutes/Mile)
1–2	1–2	15
2–3	2–2.5	12–15
4–6	2.5–3	12
7–8	3–4	12
9–10	4–5	12

TOO MUCH OF A GOOD THING: There is such a thing as too much exercise. In female marathoners and biathletes, for example, it is not uncommon for menstruation to cease. The cessation of menstruation means less estrogen, which leads to a decrease in calcium absorption, thereby increasing the risk of bone loss.

In studies conducted at the University of California, San Francisco, women who exercised to the degree they experienced amenorrhea (interruption in menstruation) were found through CT scan examinations to have lost bone mass. As is so often the case, the evidence is not absolute (other factors might also be significant), but it appears that amenorrhea puts one at a very real risk of significant bone loss.

Obviously, this is a problem in only a small portion of the population. However, if you are an avid long-distance runner or some other variety of exercise aficionado and you stop menstruating, you might be well advised to limit your training to the extent that your normal menstrual rhythms return.

Products for the Osteoporosis Patient

As with some of the treatments described in Chapter 2, you will find devices in this section that are not appropriate for your particular condition. Just as surgery isn't necessary for every osteoporosis sufferer, so, too, relatively few patients will ever require a walker or crutches. Approach the aids discussed in the following pages with a careful eye to your needs, and you will no doubt find some that will make your life easier.

You will also find a great deal of advice about selecting and using everyday items, keeping in mind the effects osteoporosis has had on your body. As an osteoporosis patient you may discover that finding a comfortable chair is harder now than it was before the pain of osteoporosis intervened. Numerous tasks assume previously unknown difficulties when a sore back makes standing and walking for prolonged periods difficult.

There are literally thousands of aids on the market that may be of use to you. Those discussed in this chapter are representative of many patients' needs and concerns. In a number of cases, no specific product is suggested, but general advice is given in the selection of everyday items. For products not generally available, the specific product is described, its approximate price cited, and a source for its purchase given.

These goods have been selected on the basis of utility and safety. However, it is recommended that you consult with your doctor or occupational therapist before adopting them, especially in the case of the more unusual items, as there may be some reason why a particular product is ill-suited to you. Often the best in-formed person on your therapeutic team is your occupational or physical therapist. The therapist will commonly discuss a possible device with your doctor. If the latter prescribes it, the cost is often tax-deductible as a medical expense. The therapist should also know where the various devices can best be obtained locally.

How to Find the Products

Most of the items cited in the following pages are generally available at department stores or hospital supply houses. In the event you have difficulty finding a particular item locally, write to the source cited and request a catalogue, price list, and, in the case of the manufacturer, the location of a store or distributor in your area where the item can be purchased. Keep in mind that mail-order firms in general charge slightly higher prices.

Be a smart shopper. Find not only the best price, but the most durable item. Durability is especially important if you will be relying on the object for your safety, or if it is something you will be using every day.

The intent of these pages is not only to direct you to helpful devices and items, but to help you make the adjustments necessary to living as normal a life as possible with your osteoporosis. You should not be afraid to be a little bit creative in thinking about the problems your osteoporosis creates for you. If you come across an item in your favorite department store that you can adapt to make your life easier, try it out, although you must always take care to consider matters of safety and good sense.

You must always think about your problem in real terms. You know your strengths and limitations better than anyone, even your doctor, so you can consider and develop solutions to your own individual problems and concerns. An essential part of dealing with your osteoporosis is anticipating trouble: if you've passed through menopause, your bones are not as strong as they were some years ago, and you are at risk of breakage. Go through your house and your everyday patterns looking for the kinds of problems enumerated earlier (see page 71) and with the concerns discussed below in mind. Safeguard yourself with a little intelligent anticipation.

Determine if some of the items cited here, especially those that can be used by more than one person, are stocked in a "loan closet" by a local hospital or health agency. If possible, it is a good idea to borrow such items to see if they work well for you. If they do, you can arrange to purchase your own. If not, return the item and don't waste your money buying it.

Personal Care: Clothing and Dressing

The selection of clothes may be more important to dealing with your osteoporosis than you realize. If you have trouble with buttons or zippers because of your osteoporosis, then you already know part of the problem. However, the issue is more than a matter of convenience.

Osteoporosis is truly a lifestyle disease: it can affect virtually all aspects of your life. For example, when selecting clothes you should be aware that items that wrap around are often easier to don than those that must be stepped into or that are put on over the head. Loose-fitting clothes and those that button in the front are also easier for many osteoporosis sufferers, especially those whose mobility is limited.

Try being more selective in thinking about how much energy each piece of an ensemble requires, and how much frustration clothes can engender on a day when your stiffness is a particular problem. You may find that some small changes in the way you select your clothes can make your life a little easier without losing your own sense of style and comfort.

Closet Hook: If you have trouble dressing, you may want to use a simple closet hook, which can be found at most hardware and houseware stores. When attached to a dowel, the closet hook can be a very versatile tool for pulling on shirts, jackets, or even trousers. In some instances, a pair of such tools may be handy in dealing with boots.

LONG-HANDLED SHOEHORN: If bending or reaching is difficult for you, a long-handled shoehorn may be the answer. Check at department and men's stores. Common lengths are 12 and 18 inches, although you may also find them as long as 24 inches.

SHOE AND BOOT REMOVER: One device that allows the removal of shoes or boots without bending is an old-fashioned boot jack. With one foot on the back of the jack to hold it steady, you insert the heel of the other shoe into the notch at the front. If you are unsure of your balance, you will be comfortable using it while seated. The book *Aids and Adaptations* (see Chapter 5) provides instructions on how one can be made simply from scrap wood.

SHOES: In selecting footwear, you would do well to consider two key issues, comfort and support: style should not be your first concern. Your shoes should fit comfortably without binding; at the same time, shoes with laces are often the best solution because they can be tied to provide a snug fit for the support you need.

Heels of more than an inch in height are not recommended as they will put undue stress on the bones and joints of the foot. For the same reason, be sure the front portions of the shoes allow for some movement of the toes within the shoe. Soft soles, too, are helpful because they cushion the feet, knees, and hips from some of the stresses of walking.

The inside of the shoe should have a soft lining for comfort. A firm heel cup is also important: your ankle will gain stability if it is prevented from rolling within the shoe. Also be sure the shoe is wide enough (look at your foot next to the shoe: if your foot appears wider, go to a wider shoe size).

Most areas have therapeutic shoe shops with knowledgeable salespeople who can fit you with the right footwear. These special shoes do cost more than regular shoes; but keep in mind it is worth getting to know a pro in the field, as he or she can help you find just the right shoes.

Personal Care: Grooming and Bathroom Products

LONG-HANDLED COMBS: If you have difficulty in reaching some portion of your hair, a long-handled comb may be helpful. A number of such devices are available (with brushes and Afro-combs as well as comb-ends). The prices range from a few dollars to as much as $20.00.

VELCRO CURLERS: These curlers require no pins or clips and so can be easily handled. They are available at most department stores.

ELEVATED TOILET SEAT: If you have sustained a hip fracture, you may find that a device which elevates the toilet seat a few inches may make trips to the bathroom easier. These toilet seats come in a variety of heights and designs, so consult your doctor or occupational therapist for recommendations.

Manufacturer: Sci-O-Tech
501 Richardson Drive
Lancaster, Pennsylvania 17603
(800) 233-0291

Sci-O-Tech makes portable raised seats that start at about $30.00. Raised seats with arms are also available in the same price range.

BATH MATS: A nonskid surface is recommended for your tub or shower. Two good candidates are a mat with suction cups on its bottom, available at most houseware stores and manufactured by Rubbermaid; or applied safety strips with adhesive backing, made by 3M. The prices are about $5.00 and $3.00, respectively. Check at department and housewares stores.

Manufacturers: Rubbermaid, Inc.
1147 Akron Road
Wooster, Ohio 44691

Minnesota Mining and Manufacturing Company
2501 Hudson Place
St. Paul, Minnesota 55119

BATHTUB RAILS: A number of different designs of bathtub rails are available; all are intended to provide a secure handhold for climbing into or out of the tub. You should consult with your doctor or occupational therapist in selecting the one best suited to your needs. Prices begin at about $25.00.

Manufacturers: Sci-O-Tech
501 Richardson Drive
Lancaster, Pennsylvania 17603
(800) 233-0291

Lumex, Inc.
100 Spence Street
Bay Shore, New York 11706
(800) 645-5272

BATH BENCHES: If lowering and raising your body into and out of the tub is difficult, a bath bench or seat may be the solution. Usually of plastic and rustproof chrome, bath seats come in a wide range of designs: with or without backs; as a transfer seat that allows entry to the tub by sliding across the bench rather than by climbing over the wall of the tub; in a variety of heights; and so on. Again, consult your doctor or occupational therapist in determining which is right for you. Prices range from under $35.00 to nearly $200.00.

Manufacturers: Sci-O-Tech
501 Richardson Drive
Lancaster, Pennsylvania 17603
(800) 233-0291

Lumex, Inc.
100 Spence Street
Bay Shore, New York 11706
(800) 645-5272

At Home: Food Preparation and Consumption

Preparing food can be a great pleasure. But to the osteoporosis patient whose energy supply is running low and whose pain quotient is approaching its zenith, it can also be utter drudgery. Since good nutrition is essential, it only makes sense to try and make food preparation as painless and pleasurable as possible.

One way to help accomplish this is to plan ahead. A few minutes invested today in reorganizing your kitchen work area may save you precious energy every time you come into the kitchen.

Consider what items you use often; keep them within easy reach of the workspace that is most comfortable for you. Think about the storage space available to you: are the cabinets or cupboards that are within easy reach filled with the objects and foodstuffs you use most often? If not, perhaps you should organize a work party of your family or friends and engineer a rearrangement.

If you have had a hip fracture, you may want to consider using a glider while preparing meals (page 129) to save steps around the kitchen.

In selecting your workspace, the height of the surface should be such that your upper arms and elbows are comfortably at your sides. This rule of thumb works whether you are standing or seated on a chair, stool, or glider. Doing the work seated will require a much lower work surface than the ordinary kitchen counter.

Time spent in the kitchen doing the ordinary and necessary gliding or walking about is the kind of exercise you should not avoid. Energy conservation is a reasonable objective, but you should approach each day or week planning to go a little farther, to do a bit more, or to stand for a little longer than you did in the days and weeks before. Such a progression tends to reduce current pain while building up your bones to prevent its recurrence.

In planning menus, the same considerations are important. Are there ways you can save steps and energy? Try cooking extra portions that can be reheated for another meal tomorrow. Cook more one-dish meals: they usually are a little less labor-intensive and can be equally tasty and nutritious. Once again, planning ahead can be very helpful, and a progressive increase in activity is bone-saving.

Microwave ovens are also a great time and energy saver. Small ones can be purchased for about $100.00, although very elaborate models range up to many hundreds of dollars.

POTS AND PANS AND OTHER CONTAINERS: Especially if you've experienced a wrist fracture, consider weight in selecting pots, pans, mixing bowls, and storage containers. Can you comfortably handle them when they are full of water or stew or other foods, or are they too heavy for you even when empty? Handles are important, too. Are the handles small or nonexistent, or can you use your entire hand to bear the weight of the container? Devices with two handles may be available and easier to use.

SPONGE MITT: If you have difficulty gripping an ordinary sponge, try a sponge mitt. You wear it like a mitten but use it as a sponge. Sponge mitts are generally available at auto parts stores and in auto sections of department stores.

WHEELED TABLE: You may find that a wheeled table or cart is useful in the kitchen, particularly when you are moving heavy items. A wheeled table can be dangerous, however, if you lean on it. The tables of various designs—some with more than one shelf, some large, some small—are generally available. Prices begin at about $20.00.

Life Around the House

CHAIRS TO WORK IN: Proper sitting position is particularly important to the osteoporosis patient who has experienced vertebral fractures, so in selecting a chair you should consider certain standards as well as your own dimensions.

If you intend to work in the chair, the backrest should reach your midback but end below your shoulder blades. The height of the chair should be such that while the entire length of your thighs rest on the seat, the heels of your feet reach the floor comfortably. The chair should support your lower back firmly.

Some chairs are available with adjustable height, swivel seats, and casters. The easy-moving items can be a hazard, though. Prices range from $100.00 up to as much as $500.00 or more.

Most office supply stores have a variety of chairs available. Try some on for size, and pick one that provides both the support you need and the comfort you like.

CHAIRS TO REST IN: For extended periods of sitting while not working, a chair should have a high back to provide support for your neck. Armrests are also important. You may find that using a thin pillow to support your lower back will make sitting more comfortable.

If you have trouble getting up from a seated position, you may want to invest in a mechanical chair that, through a spring or other mechanism, can assist in levering you out of the chair. Prices vary greatly but tend to be high, so be sure to consult with your doctor before purchasing the item: the cost of the chair may be tax deductible if the doctor recommends its purchase.

Manufacturers: Sci-O-Tech
501 Richardson Drive
Lancaster, Pennsylvania 17603
(800) 233-0291

Ortho-Kinetics, Inc.
P.O. Box 436
Waukesha, Wisconsin 53186

BEDS AND MATTRESSES: A firm mattress is important: more than a few patients have reported that a switch from a soft, sagging mattress to a firm one was the difference between back pain and none at all.

A bed board underneath the mattress is also helpful. A sheet of 1/2 inch plywood will suffice, although specially made bed boards are commercially available.

BEDDING: If you don't already, use fitted sheets. They will save you time and labor in making and remaking the bed, putting less strain on your back.

PILLOWS: Do not use more than one under your head. A specially designed contoured pillow may help you keep your head in correct alignment with your body while sleeping. Sometimes called a cervical pillow, it has a hollow at its center for your head and ridges around the edges to support your neck. Such pillows can be found at department stores or purchased from many mail-order sources. Prices are usually under $20.00.

Manufacturer: Body Care, Inc.
121 East 24th Street
New York, New York 10010
(212) 673-2955

BED CADDY: If you are bedridden for a considerable period of time, you may find a sort of "bed saddlebag" useful for holding reading and writing materials, glasses, or other small objects. Bed caddies can easily be made from a strong, durable material, although some are commercially available.

LONG-HANDLED DUSTPAN: This tool will be particularly useful if you have trouble bending and reaching the floor. Again, most housewares stores carry them for about $5.00.

POCKET APRONS: You may find an apron with pockets can simplify numerous tasks around the house, whether it is simply neatening up or pursuing a hobby or household task. The pockets enable you easily to tote small objects with you and to keep them accessible and organized. You will find household aprons in most department stores; for heavier objects and sturdier wear, you may want to try a carpenter's apron, generally available at hardware stores. Be careful, however, not to load yourself down so that your balance is affected by what you are carrying.

READING AIDS: The osteoporosis sufferer who remains in the same position for a prolonged period will likely become stiff and uncomfortable. As a result, a bookstand is recommended to allow the hands and arms to rest while reading.

A number of different bookstands of different designs are available. In the publication *Aids and Adaptations* (see Chapter 5), plans are provided for the construction of a wooden reading stand. One commercially made stand costs less than $30.00, can be used in bed or in a chair, and adjusts to a variety of angles.

Manufacturer: Replogle Globes
1901 North Narragansett Avenue
Chicago, Illinois 60639-3885

REACHING DEVICES: If your range of motion has become limited—or if you are confined to bed—then a pair of tongs may be helpful to you. There are a great variety of models on the market, some of which are expensive, some well designed, some not. Check at hardware stores.

You may find it handy to have more than one pair: one in the kitchen, one in the pantry, one by the bed.

WORK SURFACES: Be sure that whatever your work surface, you can sit comfortably with your back straight and your shoulders relaxed. If your desk is too low, you will find yourself stooping. For typing, it is recommended that the typewriter be located so that your elbows are at right angles while at the keyboard.

For reading or writing, you may find that a work surface that is slanted toward you works best. Artists' drafting tables are generally available with adjustable slant tops, but a simpler, less expensive solution may be simply to prop up a board with books or a box.

RAMPS: If you are wheelchair-bound or have great difficulty with stairs at the entrance to your home, a ramp may be a suitable solution. There are plans available (see Chapter 5, *Aids and Adaptations*) for a contractor to follow.

Key concerns are that the pitch of the ramp not exceed one inch of rise per twelve inches of run; that there be a railing on unprotected sides; and that the surface of the ramp be made of a nonskid material.

STAIRWAY LIFTS: Devices are available that will deliver you (and, in some configurations, your wheelchair as well) up or down a flight of stairs. These devices are expensive (generally over $1,000.00, plus installation cost), but some can be leased on a rental/option-to-buy agreement.

Manufacturers: R.J. Mobility Systems, Inc.
715 South Fifth Avenue
Maywood, Illinois 60153

Econol Stairway Lift Corporation
2513 Center Street
Cedar Falls, Iowa 50613

In the Office

DESK ORGANIZERS: As in the kitchen, organization is crucial at your desk. A great variety of equipment is available that can help you keep the office tools and supplies you need within easy reach, to minimize the amount of walking and twisting and turning and reaching required of you.

Desktop caddies for writing utensils and other small paraphernalia are sold at most office supply stores, as are stationery and paper racks that can be placed on your desktop or nearby. File cabinets on rollers are also generally available; storing your most active files in them can save you heavy pulling while bent over, an unsafe maneuver for the patient with osteoporosis.

PORTABLE PHONES:　A portable phone may be very handy. If you are wheelchair-bound or rely on crutches or a cane for mobility, you will appreciate not having to rush to the phone when it rings, as you can keep the phone with you in a shoulder pack or hanging from your chair.

WRITING MATERIALS:　It is often easier on the back, neck, and shoulders if your writing surface is slanted slightly. A variety of lap desks may be useful, too, if you are bedridden or choose to attend to your correspondence in bed.

If you have difficulty grasping pencils or pens, you may wish to use larger diameter writing utensils or to build up those you have with foam or rubber. Foam curlers into which you insert the pen or pencil are one possible solution.

Orthotics

The Greek word *orthosis* means "to make straight"; combined with *ped* as in pediatrics, we have orthopedics, the branch of medicine that originally was concerned with straightening children's twisted spines. Today, the discipline is more wide-ranging: an orthopedic surgeon is a specialist in bone and joint surgery for both children and adults. The word *orthosis* also produced the name orthotist, or one who makes braces and splints. Orthotists often begin their professional lives as occupational or physical therapists.

BACK BRACES:　In the case of osteoporosis, orthopedic appliances are an occasional weapon of control, particularly for fractures that cause acute and severe pain that doesn't subside in a week or so. In such a circumstance, a brace may be prescribed by your doctor or orthopedic surgeon and made for you by an orthotist. Back braces are to be regarded in virtually all cases as a temporary measure. You should expect to spend less and less time in the brace as the pain recedes and eventually to abandon it altogether.

Orthotics are best custom made. Plastic and foam are most commonly used; Velcro fastenings are a frequent element. A back support will often have shoulder straps and will be carefully fitted for you. It is important that such braces be used only with the guidance of your doctor or orthopedic surgeon. The cost of orthotics, when prescribed by a doctor, is tax deductible.

Ambulation Aids

CANES: Canes are particularly useful for patients recovering from hip fractures. The cane is held in the hand opposite the affected side.

Canes can be purchased from hospital equipment suppliers. There are a variety of handles available, but it is recommended that whatever its source, the cane be fitted with a rubber tip for maximum stability. The tip must be a minimum of 1 1/2 inches in diameter. Most hospital supply stores carry them at under $4.00 each.

Manufacturers: Guardian Products Co., Inc.
780 East Street
P.O. Box 549
Simi Valley, California 93062

Guardian Products Co., Inc.
3043 Fleetbrook Drive
P.O. Box 16967
Memphis, Tennessee 38116

Guardian Products Co., Inc.
16 Passaic Avenue
P.O. Box 1325
Fairfield, New Jersey 07006

As usual, it is very important that your cane be selected under the guidance of your doctor or physical therapist. Height, handle, and weight are among the other concerns that must be considered.

CRUTCHES: Crutches come in a much greater variety of configurations than canes, and, again, it is crucial that your doctor or physical therapist be consulted in their selection. The height must be properly adjusted to your size and the handgrips properly suited; there are a multitude of designs for different needs and uses, and prices vary enormously. Be sure you get crutches that will help you the most.

Handgrips are especially important if your wrists are affected by osteoporosis. Forearm platforms may be useful: they allow you to distribute your weight along the length of your forearm as you walk, rather than resting it on the hands or wrists. Prices range from under $20.00 to over $100.00.

Manufacturers: Lumex, Inc.
100 Spence Street
Bay Shore, New York 11706
(800) 645-5272

Guardian Products Co., Inc.
780 East Street
P.O. Box 549
Simi Valley, California 93062

Guardian Products Co., Inc.
3043 Fleetbrook Drive
P.O. Box 16967
Memphis, Tennessee 38116

Guardian Products Co., Inc.
16 Passaic Avenue
P.O. Box 1325
Fairfield, New Jersey 07006

CANE CLIPS: If you rely on your crutches or cane to get around, you will understand how useful "cane parkers" can be. Several varieties are available, including those that can be permanently attached to your favorite chair or bedside table and those that go with you on your cane wherever you go. Prices vary for the many different designs but should be less than $2.50 for the mobile clips and about $1.00 for those that remain on individual pieces and furniture.

WALKERS, GLIDERS, AND WHEELCHAIRS: Walkers are for those people who need more stability than a cane can offer; wheelchairs are for patients whose lower extremities are so severely affected that walking is no longer possible. Gliders fit somewhere between: they are wheeled chairs, but they rely on the legs and feet to provide locomotion.

It is imperative that you get your doctor's or physical therapist's guidance before selecting a walker, glider, or wheelchair.

Manufacturers: Lumex, Inc.
100 Spence Street
Bay Shore, New York 11706

Sci-O-Tech
501 Richardson Drive
Lancaster, Pennsylvania 17603

Gliders are also made by Lumex, as well as by:

Activeaid
501 East Tin Street
Redwood Falls, Minnesota 56283

An aid to movement for traveling greater distances is a motorized unit. Power wheelchairs are available, as are scooter-like devices with swivel seats. They fit into the trunk of a car and most run on a 12-volt battery.

Prices are typically more than $1,000, but the scooter-like units are quite useful for people who are not wheelchair-bound but who have difficulty standing for extended periods or walking distances. One typical model is the Portascoot.

Manufacturer: E. F. Brewer Company
13901 Main Street
P.O. Box 159
Menomonee Falls, Wisconsin 53051-0159
(800) 558-8777

A second model is made by Amigo.

Manufacturer: Amigo Sales, Inc.
6693 Dixie Highway
Bridgeport, Michigan 48722-0402
(800) 248-9131

Away from Home

BELT PACKS: Whether you are going out for a short jaunt in the park or taking a longer trip, you may find that a belt pack will enable you to carry small, useful objects without encumbering your hands. Belt packs and small knapsacks can be found in most sporting goods shops. Prices begin at about $5.00.

LUGGAGE CARRIER: When you are traveling, luggage caddies can make carrying your baggage a great deal easier, relieving stress on your back. In selecting one for your use, be sure the carrier folds up conveniently and adjusts to fit your baggage. A number of different designs are generally available at department stores or luggage shops. Prices range from about $15.00 to $50.00.

SEAT CUSHION: If your back troubles you or if you are at the wheel of your car for long periods, a cushion that supports your lower back may make you more comfortable. Available at many auto supply stores, they generally sell for under $15.00.

Mail-Order Source: Medical SELF-CARE Catalog
P.O. Box 999
Point Reyes, California 94956

WIDE-ANGLE MIRROR: If you find that your osteoporosis limits the motion of your upper body to a degree that you are not confident of your ability to see behind you, a wide-angle mirror may be helpful. It slides over your standard mirror and has a day/night adjustment. Many different models are available at auto parts stores for approximately $10.00.

CHAPTER 5

Selected Print
and
Audiovisual Materials

If what you learned in the previous chapters of this book has made you want to know more, there is an extensive library of print and audiovisual materials available to you.

The intent of this closing chapter is to provide you with specific sources for further information. The first section presents the available publications, ranging from pamphlets that require only minutes to read to complex, full-length reference works. The concluding section lists audiovisual materials, including films and videotapes.

Both the print and audiovisual sections of this chapter are divided, in turn, into subsections. The first subsection includes materials that offer general information about osteoporosis. The second includes sources that emphasize the physical and emotional management of the ailment; the third focuses on medications, the fourth on surgery.

If you want to know more about your osteoporosis, the odds are that you will find a suitable source of information listed in the following pages.

Print
Materials

Many of the publications listed here are available for purchase at your local bookstore or can be borrowed from your library.

Others, however, in particular specialty pamphlets and booklets from nonprofit or federally funded foundations or organizations, are not likely to be on your bookstore or library shelves. Usually these publications are available by mail for free or for a nominal charge.

When you come across references to such publications in the following pages, you will also find the addresses of the relevant organization along with the entry that describes the books or pamphlet in question. The phone number and other pertinent order information are also included.

This chapter does not attempt to provide a complete list of every available publication but rather discusses a representative selection of materials that constitute the best and most valuable.

General Information

Calcium: You Never Outgrow Your Need For It
Rosemont, Illinois: National Dairy Council, 1986. Unpaginated. FREE

As you can tell from its title, this pamphlet is concerned with calcium. It begins with a simple test ("Have You Fed Your Bones Lately?"), in which the reader is asked to check off the number of times on the previous day he or she ate cheese, collard greens, ice cream, pizza, or other calcium-containing foods.

The test is an easy way to raise the consciousness of those unaware of the need for calcium and unfamiliar with which foods contain it. While this pamphlet won't offer the reader of this book new information, it might be of value in alerting others less well informed to an important issue. It mentions osteoporosis only in passing. It is especially recommended for those under age forty.

The pamphlet is available from the National Dairy Council, 6300 North River Road, Rosemont, Illinois 60018. Telephone: (312) 696-1020.

The Menopause Years
Washington, D.C.: The American College of Obstetricians and Gynecologists, 1984. Unpaginated.
FREE

This small booklet takes a no-nonsense yet positive approach to menopause. The emphasis is on the possibilities as well as the facts. For example, a short section on sexuality goes this way:

> A woman's sexuality does not have to be affected by menopause. If a woman had regular sexual relations before menopause, she will probably remain active throughout and after menopause. Difficulties with sex around the time of menopause may be related to the effects of the loss of estrogen. Intercourse can be painful. Dryness of the vagina can be treated with estrogen creams or lubricating jellies. With regular sexual relations the lining of the vagina retains its natural elasticity and becomes lubricated naturally. Longer foreplay also enhances lubrication.
>
> Sexual relations often become more desirable at this stage in life. A woman and her partner have more time for each other and often find this brings them closer together. They are also more experienced sexually and know how to please each other. Some women may feel relieved and find that they have sexual relations more often.

Other issues discussed include cessation of menstruation, early menopause, hot flushes, vaginal changes, emotional aspects, and the pros and cons of estrogen replacement therapy. Although osteoporosis is not discussed per se, this accessible pamphlet makes informative and reassuring reading for women approaching or experiencing menopause.

Osteoporosis
Park Ridge, Illinois: American Academy of Orthopaedic
    Surgeons, 1986. Unpaginated.
FREE

This brief but to-the-point pamphlet identifies osteoporosis, explains its consequences, and discusses the importance of calcium, vitamin D, and exercise. It also briefly identifies detection methods and offers suggestions for the prevention of further bone loss.

This publication is available upon request from the American Academy of Orthopaedic Surgeons, 222 South Prospect Avenue, Park Ridge, Illinois 60068-4058. Telephone: (312) 825-7186. Given its brevity, its value is limited largely to those unfamiliar with osteoporosis; it might best be used as a handout to introduce the uninitiated to the basic facts of the ailment.

Osteoporosis: Brittle Bones and the Calcium Crisis
Mayes, Kathleen
Santa Barbara, California: Pennant Books, 1986. 176 pages.
$8.95

A sensible overview of osteoporosis, its risks, and related factors, this book is strongest when talking about what you can do yourself. Described as a health and nutrition guide, the book devotes many pages to dietary aspects, including more than a dozen pages of food tables.

Osteoporosis: Cause, Treatment, Prevention
National Institute of Arthritis and Musculoskeletal and
  Skin Diseases
Bethesda, Maryland: National Institutes of Health, 1984. 38
  pages.
FREE

This booklet is the result of the 1984 National Institutes of Health Consensus Development Conference on Osteoporosis. It was revised slightly in 1986 to incorporate new research.

Written with the layperson in mind, the booklet is a readable and well-organized introduction to the problem of osteoporosis. It speaks both to those with the ailment and to women concerned that they may develop it in later life.

Especially useful are food charts of some calcium-rich foods, a handy aid to planning meals high in calcium.

To receive a single copy, send a business-sized (4″ × 9 1/2″ minimum), self-addressed envelope with $.50 postage to: Osteoporosis Booklet, NIAMS/National Institutes of Health, Box

AMS, Bethesda, Maryland 20892. Larger quantities are also available. Send $2.00 for postage and handling for ten copies, $5.00 for twenty-five, or $10.00 for fifty. Make checks payable to "AMS Clearinghouse." Organizations may reprint all or portions of the booklet for their own use without permission.

Osteoporosis: How to Prevent the Brittle-Bone Disease
Smith, Wendy, in consultation with Dr. Stanton H. Cohn
New York, New York: A Fireside Book, Simon & Schuster, Inc.,
   1985. 142 pages.
$5.95

This overview of osteoporosis is distinguished in two ways: first, it contains more than thirty pages of very specific menus and recipes; second, it is written with wit and intelligence.

The book tells you what you need to know without weighing you down with more than you need. And the author has a sense of humor, too. For example, in discussing dietary sources of calcium, she informs us, "[S]hould you suddenly find a butcher shop that sells alligator meat on a regular basis, your calcium worries are over. One three-and-a-half ounce pieces contains 1,231 mg. of calcium! Don't try nibbling on your handbag, though; the skin isn't where the calcium is."

The menus are organized by weeks. There are specific foods recommended, meal-by-meal, day-by-day for a four-week plan. The recipes are easy to follow and wide-ranging (from Miso Soup to Cornbread and Spinach Squares), and all cite both calcium and caloric contents for each ingredient.

Osteoporosis: Your Head Start on the Prevention and
   Treatment of Brittle Bones
Fardon, David F., M.D.
New York, New York: Macmillan Publishing Company, 1985.
   276 pages.
$15.95

Though written with the layperson in mind, this is a lengthy and detailed discussion of osteoporosis. If you are interested in a few key nuggets of information, then *Osteoporosis: Cause, Treatment, Prevention* from the National Institute of Arthritis and Musculoskeletal and Skin Diseases is probably for you (it's only thirty-eight pages long). On the other hand, if you are interested in the whole story well told, try this one.

Fardon gives the facts—he is an orthopedic surgeon at the University of Missouri Medical Center—but he also offers a generous amount of history and background. This anecdote recounted in Chapter 3 of his book suggests his wide-ranging approach:

The solution to the mystery of bone growth began in 1736, when a London printer invited a young surgeon, John Belchier, to dinner. Belchier noticed a ruddy, red staining in the bones of the roast pig served by his host. Fortunately for science, Belchier was not too polite to inquire about the discolored bones. The printer revealed that he had been feeding bran to his pigs. The bran had been soaked with madder, a plant whose roots and berries serve as sources of red dye. Belchier fed animals madder and then examined their bones. If he stopped giving the animals madder and fed them regular food for a while before they were killed, their bones did not look red from the outside. Cut bones, however, showed a red layer beneath the surface. Belchier reasoned that bones, like trees, grew by depositing new layers around the outside. He had discovered a way to measure that growth.

A readable and informative book for the person who wants a thorough knowledge of osteoporosis.

Osteoporosis: What It Is, How to Prevent It, How to Stop It
Kamen, Betty, Ph.D., and Si Kamen
New York, New York: Pinnacle Books, 1984. 222 pages.
$3.50

Although thoroughly researched (there are seventy pages of notes and appendices), this book wanders occasionally into uncertain territory: the authors warn against underarm spray that contains aluminum, for example.

The book's most useful aspect is its collection of recipes.

Preventing Osteoporosis
Washington, D.C.: The American College of Obstetricians
    and Gynecologists, 1984. Unpaginated.
FREE

This booklet offers a quick, no-nonsense introduction to the rudiments of preventing osteoporosis. It explains the risk factors, the basics of bone and its metabolism, and the nature of osteoporosis. It covers the key points in a brief but surprisingly thorough manner.

Also contained in this booklet is a two-page illustrated chart of approximately thirty common foods, citing both the fat and calcium content in a typical serving. Other issues discussed include estrogen replacement therapy and the importance of regular gynecological exams and attendant tests.

Although the information in this pamphlet will be familiar to those who have read this book, the pamphlet would be of considerable use either for discussion groups or as an easily absorbed introduction for younger women who feel unable to commit a substantial block of time to becoming familiar with the basics of prevention.

Stand Tall! The Informed Woman's Guide to Preventing Osteoporosis
Notelowitz, Morris D., and Marsha Ware
New York, New York: Bantam Books, Inc., 1982. 208 pages.
$7.95

Despite its subtitle, this book is aimed at women with osteoporosis as well as those concerned with its avoidance.

The book is well illustrated, with more than thirty photos, drawings, charts, and graphs. Divided into numerous chapters and subsections, *Stand Tall!* lends itself to browsing as well as to cover-to-cover review. By using the index or various headings, one can find a few hundred words on most of the important areas of concern that summarize the subject at hand.

For example, in a section titled "Risk Factors You Cannot Control," there is this discussion of genetic factors.

Get out the family album. Your heredity plays an important role in determining the amount of bone you have at maturity and your rate of bone loss with age. The best evidence for this comes from studies of twins. Identical twins have more closely matched bone mass than fraternal twins, and both types of twins are more closely matched than other siblings. We also know that many, if not most, women with osteoporosis have a family history of the disorder.

Therefore you will want to know your family history. If your grandmother, mother, aunt, or sister has osteoporosis, you are well-advised to consider yourself at high risk. Nevertheless, lack of a family history of the disorder should not give you false confidence, since many other factors can influence your bone mass and your overall risk of osteoporosis.

This book is a sound overview of our knowledge of osteoporosis. However, as research advances continue, the hard science in it is gradually becoming dated.

Understanding Calcium and Osteoporosis
American Allergy Association
Menlo Park, California: Allergy Publication Group, 1987.
  16 pages.
FREE

Despite its brevity, the booklet covers most of the important aspects of calcium's role in the body and the nature of osteoporosis, its treatment, and prevention. Risk factors are discussed at length.

While little is said about the course of osteoporosis, much good dietary advice is offered. The reader will get a clear understanding of calcium's importance and specific guidance in how to go about getting enough from dietary and other sources.

It is available from the Allergy Publication Group, P.O. Box 640, Menlo Park, California 94026. Telephone: (415) 322-1663.

It is available at special prices for bulk purposes and would be suitable for groups requiring a practical, easy-to-read primer on the importance of calcium to women, with or without osteoporosis.

Understanding Paget's Disease

Bethesda, Maryland: National Institute of Arthritis and
   Musculoskeletal and Skin Diseases, 1985. Unpaginated.
FREE

Paget's disease is, in a sense, the reverse of osteoporosis: it is a chronic ailment of the skeleton characterized by the accumulation of too much bone mass. The result of Paget's disease is not unlike osteoporosis, however, as the bones grow weak and may become deformed or fracture.

Also known as osteitis deformans, Paget's disease occurs when too much bone tissue is broken down and in response the body increases the rate at which new tissue is formed. The new bone is disordered, in some cases soft, and not as strong as normal bone.

Disease activity in patients with Paget's disease is usually localized. The spine, skull, pelvis, thighs, and lower legs are most often affected. Although the ailment is progressive, it is asymptomatic (that is, without symptoms) in most patients. When the ailment makes itself known, the symptoms are usually pain and a warm sensation in the affected area. Lab tests of the blood and urine, as well as x-rays and bone scans, are the usual means of confirming the diagnosis.

This pamphlet explains the basic facts of the ailment, including its treatment (calcitonin and other drugs) and its likely course. It is available free of charge from the National Arthritis and Musculoskeletal and Skin Diseases Clearinghouse, National Institutes of Health, Box AMS, Bethesda, Maryland 20892. Telephone: (301) 468-3235.

If you suffer from Paget's disease, you or your physician may wish to be in contact with the Paget's Disease Foundation, Box 2772, Brooklyn, New York 11202.

Physical and Emotional Management

Accent On Living Buyer's Guide: 1988–1989 Edition
Bloomington, Illinois: Cheever Publishing, Inc., 1988. 152 pages.
$10.00

This is a sourcebook for products. It offers no assessments or descriptions of products; but if you know what you want, you are more than likely to find a source for it here.

Categorized by problem area (among the thirty-three areas are Dressing, Drinking, Eating, Education, and Exercising), each section is broken down into subcategories: the subheads under Exercising, for example, include Bicycle exerciser, Exerciser (hand), Exerciser (passive), Mats, Therapy balls, Trimcycle, Weights (wheelchair use), and Weights (wrist and ankle). Following each subhead is the name of one or more manufacturers, whose addresses are to be found in a separate section of the book.

The volume also includes the addresses of numerous organizations, publications, and service groups, as well as numerous advertisements. It is published by Accent (page 86).

Aids and Adaptations
Occupational Therapy Department, British Columbia Division
Toronto: The Arthritis Society.
$2.50

Although intended for arthritis patients, this publication may be of considerable use to osteoporosis patients.

Subtitled "A Collection of Designs," this book contains a number of useful items, including a plan for constructing an entrance ramp and a wooden reading stand. It also offers valuable advice on techniques for dressing, eating, grooming, and other daily activities, as well as suggestions on how to make, easily and inexpensively, numerous tools and aids to accomplish everyday tasks more easily.

The pamphlet is available from The Arthritis Society, 250 Bloor Street, Suite 401, Toronto, Ontario M4W 3P2, Canada. Telephone: (416) 967-1914. You will find this a very practical and useful book if your osteoporosis interferes with your ability to do many ordinary tasks.

The All-American Guide to Calcium-rich Foods
Rosemont, Illinois: National Dairy Council, 1986. Unpaginated.
FREE

This pamphlet consists largely of food tables listing dietary sources of calcium. "Primary calcium sources" are milk products; "secondary sources" are meats, fruits and vegetables, grains, or combination foods. There is also a discussion of calcium supplements. Each table includes the number of milligrams of calcium per serving.

This pamphlet's value is as a convenient reference for calcium-rich foods. It would be helpful as a handout for use in group discussions.

It is available from the National Dairy Council, 6300 North River Road, Rosemont, Illinois 60018. Telephone: (312) 696-1020.

Coping With Stress: Making Stress Work for You
Atlanta: The Arthritis Foundation
Catalog No.: 9326
FREE

Although this booklet addresses the subject of stress and its interrelationship with arthritis, the osteoporosis patient may well find it of value. It identifies signs of stress and offers strategies for reducing it.

Coping With Stress discusses the importance of accepting what you cannot change. It also offers specific relaxation techniques. One technique, for example, involves the use of mental pictures. "Light a candle," the booklet suggests, "and focus your attention on the flame [for] a few minutes. Then close your eyes and watch the image of the flame for a minute or two."

This booklet is a useful tool not only for the osteoporosis sufferer but for anyone who finds that the strains and pressures of everyday life have a harmful impact on his or her physical and mental well-being.

An Easier Way: Handbook for the Elderly and Handicapped
Sargeant, Jean V.
New York: Walker Publishing, 1982. 218 pages.
$12.95

This books contains over 200 suggestions of methods and devices to help people with functional limitations carry out day-to-day tasks and activities. Subjects covered include cooking and eating, dressing, bathroom aids, mobility, and sleeping.

The 1987 Educational Resource Guide on Osteoporosis
Quinn, Phyllis, M.Ed.
Alexandria, Virginia: American Physical Therapy Association, 1987. Unpaginated.
$3.00

If you still have a desire to know more, order a copy of this publication. It lists resources for physical therapists, other health professionals, articles, audiovisual materials, books, organizations, and research.

A number of the sources and publications cited in the publication can be found in this volume; however, if you are interested in more technical publications (journal articles or academic books), the bibliographic sections in this guide will be of value to you.

The Wheelchair Gourmet: A Cookbook for the Disabled
New York: Beaufort Books, 1981. 219 pages.
$8.95

A useful guide, including recipes, for people who have trouble maneuvering in the kitchen. There are hints on standard cooking procedures and on gadgets for people whose hands or arms are weakened by disease or who are in wheelchairs.

There is some nutritional advice as well. However, because the advice is based principally on experience rather than medical evidence, it should not override your doctor's recommendations.

Medications

Advice for the Patient, Volume 2.
Rockville, Maryland: The U.S. Pharmacopoeia Convention, Inc., 1985.
$23.95

Organized by generic name, this standard reference manual identifies the use and side effects and offers other information about over-the-counter and prescription medications.

It can be purchased from the U.S. Pharmacopeia Convention, Inc., 12601 Twinbrook Parkway, Rockville, Maryland 20852. Many libraries will have this volume in their reference collections.

The Essential Guide to Prescription Drugs
Long, James W., M.D.
New York: Harper & Row, 1987. 933 pages.
$12.95

Written for a lay audience, this is a handy reference on prescription drugs. Each generic drug has a separate entry, which includes, among other information, the benefits and risks of each; the dosage; the side effects; the effects on pregnancy, breast feeding, and ailments; and advice on precautions regarding other medications, alcohol and driving.

Estrogen Replacement Therapy
Washington, D.C.: The American College of Obstetricians and Gynecologists, 1986. 6 pages.
FREE

This technical bulletin may be useful to those patients who feel they must know everything possible about the medication they are taking. Although it was written for physicians, it can be understood by the layperson if read with reference to a medical dictionary.

Available from the American College of Obstetricians and Gynecologists, 600 Maryland Avenue, SW, Suite 300 East, Washington, D.C. 20024-2588.

The Food and Drug Interaction Guide
Morgan, Brian L., Ph.D.
New York, New York: Simon and Schuster, 1986. 335 pages. $10.95

Organized by generic drugs, this book offers specific information and guidance regarding the interactions in your body when you take certain drugs.

In the entry on the diuretic spironolactone, for example, the author warns of the dangers of a calcium deficiency. He also explains the risks of potassium toxicity in this way:

Spironolactone reduces the normal excretion of potassium, so in some people, particularly those with diseased kidneys that cannot excrete potassium very effectively, potassium levels could conceivably build up in the body, leading to potassium toxicity (hyperkalemia).

Prevention and Treatment: While you are on spironolactone, you should not be taking potassium supplements, nor should a diet rich in potassium be consumed. Potassium-rich foods include tomato juice, lentils, dried apricots, asparagus, bananas, peanut butter, chicken, almonds, and milk.

The interactions of more than 300 generic drugs (which represent more than a thousand brand name drugs) are discussed. Both over-the-counter and prescription drugs are included.

Physicians' Desk Reference, 42nd Edition
Oradell, New Jersey: Medical Economics Co., 1988. $34.95

This annual publication is the standard reference your doctor uses to get the basic information available about the medications he or she prescribes. Although much of it may be unintelligible to the layperson, the entries concerning drugs you take on a maintenance basis may be well worth reading. However, given its cost and technical nature, it is advised you make reference to the book in your local library.

A section of actual-size color photographs of the capsules and pills is a useful feature of the book.

The Pill Box
The Food and Drug Book Co., Inc.
New York: Bantam Books, 1985. 196 pages.
$3.95

This reference work consists of a brief introduction to and more detailed description of several hundred generic drugs. The profiles of the individual drugs constitute the bulk of the book; the book's intent is to provide for the layperson some of the basic information the *Physicians' Desk Reference* (see previous entry) offers to the medical professional.

Like the PDR, the book includes a section of color photographs of commonly used capsules and pills.

Surgery

Daily Activities After Your Hip Surgery
Platt, Janet Verner, et al.
Rockville, Maryland: The American Occupational Therapy
    Association, Inc., 1986. 18 pages.
$5.20

Written and compiled by the staff of the Division of Occupational Therapy, Georgetown University Hospital, this booklet is intended to guide the patient recovering from hip surgery through the adjustment necessary to the disability. Through the use of text and clear, easy-to-understand drawings, the reader is advised about the do's and don'ts of sitting, using a walker, showering, using the toilet and bathtub, sleeping, getting in and out of a car, dressing, and other daily activities.

This publication is available from the American Occupational Therapy Association, Inc., Products Division, 1383 Piccard Drive, P.O. Box 1725, Rockville, Maryland 1725.

Orthopaedics
Park Ridge, Illinois: American Academy of Orthopaedic
    Surgeons, 1986. Unpaginated.
FREE

This pamphlet explains what an orthopedic surgeon is, what the qualifications are, and common problems these professionals are trained to address. It also explains diagnostic techniques, the kinds of procedures practiced, and the rehabilitation process.

This publication is available upon request from the American Academy of Orthopaedic Surgeons, 222 South Prospect Avenue, Park Ridge, Illinois 60068-4058. Telephone: (312) 825-7186. However, given its brevity, its value is limited. It might best be used as a handout to provide a basic profile of the orthopedist.

Audiovisual Materials

This section presents audiovisual materials recommended for patient and professional use. The materials are listed in alphabetical order by title and are divided into the same subject divisions used in the print materials section.

Many public, professional, and medical libraries will have some or all of these materials available for rental. Check with the reference librarian at your local library to help you find the nearest source. In all cases, mail-order sources are cited in the entry in the event you are unable to find them in your community.

General Information

An Aging Process—Osteoporosis
Available from: Fairview General Audio-Visuals, 18101 Lorain
  Avenue, Cleveland, Ohio 44111-5656. (216) 476-7054.
Film or videotape
$450 (film purchase)
$65 (film rental)
$295 (videotape purchase)
$60 (videotape rental)

This film is intended to help nurses, dietitians, and community
health workers develop an understanding of how osteoporosis
affects the body in order to help in its diagnosis and prevention.
Recommended for caregivers rather than osteoporosis sufferers.

Brittle Bones
Available from: Filmmakers Library, 133 East 58th Street,
  New York, New York 10022. (212) 355-6545.
16-minute film or videotape
$450 (film purchase)
$400 (video purchase)
$50 (film rental)

This film describes the clinical details of osteoporosis but also
offers a human story in the person of eighty-eight-year-old Lin-
dy Frazier, a women in a wheelchair for almost fifty years who
regained mobility through exercise and fluoride treatments.
  Brittle Bones was produced by the Canadian Broadcasting
Corporation.

Brittle With Age: The Unnecessary Tragedy of Osteoporosis
Available from: Melpomene Institute for Women's Health
  Research, 2125 East Hennepin Avenue, Minneapolis,
  Minnesota 55413. (612) 378-0545.
23-minute videotape
$300.00 (purchase)
$50.00 (rental)
$35.00 (rental to nonprofit organization)

The primary emphasis is on the personal experience of osteoporosis patients. The film features discussions with patients and doctors about the ailment, along with its diagnosis and treatment.

In addition, there is a section on prevention, in which exercise, calcium intake, and estrogen therapy are discussed.

A short pamphlet is available to accompany the tape which summarizes much of the basic information.

Nutrition for Today's Woman
Available from: Professional Research, Inc., 930 Pitner,
   Evanston, Illinois 60202. (800) 421-2363.
12½-minute film or videotape
$295.00

This film provides a brief overview of good eating habits. Although not aimed specifically at the osteoporosis patient, sensible advice is offered regarding appropriate and inappropriate foods, weight control, and alcohol and caffeine use. The importance of calcium is another issue presented, as is the importance of exercise.

Osteoporosis
Available from: Soundwords, Inc., 56-11 217th Street, Bayside,
   New York 11364
Audiotape
$12.95

A tape in the "Doctor Talks to You . . ." series, this audiotape features Joseph M. Lane, M.D., Professor of Orthopedic Surgery at the Cornell University Medical College and Chief, Metabolic Bone Disease, at the Hospital for Special Surgery in New York City.

His talk offers a basic introduction to the causes, symptoms, and treatment of osteoporosis.

Osteoporosis: NIH Consensus
Available from: American Journal of Nursing Company, Rental
   Library, c/o Mediatech, 110 West Hubbard Street, Chicago,
   Illinois 60610. (800) 621-7018; in Illinois, (312) 828-1146.
Order Numbers: 9004V (rental); L9004J (purchase)
48-minute videotape
$60.00 (rental)
$350.00 (purchase)

Although aimed primarily at nurses involved in the care of
osteoporosis sufferers, this film presents a variety of nationally
known experts on osteoporosis talking about the ailment at the
1983 NIH Consensus Development Conference on Osteoporosis.
The format is question-and-answer: orthopedists, gynecologists,
nutritionists, and other experts are asked questions. The topics
they discuss include risk groups; causes and symptoms; the role
of therapies like estrogen, supplemental calcium, and vitamin D;
and prevention and treatment through diet and exercise.

The bulk of this information is covered in many publications;
some is now dated. However, for people unable or unwilling to
read about osteoporosis, this film will help provide a basic
understanding of the ailment and its current treatment.

Physical and Emotional Management

Activity and Exercise
Available from: Dartmouth-Hitchcock Medical Center, Arthritis
   Center, Hanover, New Hampshire 03756. (603) 646-7700.
51 slides, audiocassette
$100.00 (purchase)
$15.00 (one-week rental)

Although designed to help arthritis patients think about their
activities—both planned exercises and normal movements—these
materials are of value to the patient with osteoporosis. The idea
is to divide the activities into three classes: activities of daily living, traditional exercises, and therapeutic exercises. The approach

is pragmatic: plan ahead, think about what will be painful for you, balance the need for a particular task with the benefit (or harm) you will get from it.

The producer recommends that the presenter of the program be a physical therapist so that he or she can answer patients' questions and direct an accompanying practice session.

No Place Like Home: Long Term Care for the Elderly
Available from: Filmmakers Library, 133 East 58th Street, New York, New York 10022. (212) 355-6545.
55-minute videotape
$445 (purchase)
$75 (rental)

Helen Hayes narrates this look at institutional home care, which argues that home care is less expensive and more desirable for the older person. The film's archival material takes us back to the origins of today's nursing home (the almshouses of the 1800s) and offers several alternatives to such institutions. Settings include New York, Appalachia, San Francisco, and England.

In conclusion, the eighty-one-year-old Ms. Hayes says, "Science has taught us to lengthen life. Now we must learn to make a longer life worth living. Older people deserve choices. For most of us, there's no place like home."

The ROM Dance: A Range of Motion Exercise and Relaxation Program
Available from: Friends of WHA-TV, Inc., Program Marketing, 821 University Avenue, Madison, Wisconsin, 53706. (608) 263-2121.
45-minute videotape, 2 audiocassettes, and 113-page accompanying text

Based on the principles of the ancient Chinese exercise T'ai-Chi Ch'uan, the ROM dance sequence and relaxation program blends joint exercises with stress-reducing relaxation.

The videotape offers an introduction to the ROM dance, including participants discussing how it has affected their daily lives. In addition, there is a demonstration of the dance sequence. The text includes a discussion of the ROM dance philosophy, illustrations of the sequence, forty-five relaxation exercises, precautions, and sample handouts for participants.

Telephone the Friends of WHA-TV for costs for purchasing or renting all or a portion of the package. Note that there is a second, less expensive price list for nonprofit organizations.

Medication

A Clinical Approach to Estrogen Replacement Therapy
Available from: Ayerst CME Library, 22 Riverview Drive, Wayne, New Jersey 07470-3191. (201) 628-8234.
Order Number: 510-0627
30-minute film or videotape
Free to physicians

This film, prepared under the auspices of a manufacturer of estrogen medications, is a presentation of guidelines for the use of estrogen replacement therapy. The participating doctors assess the risk profiles of three patients deficient in estrogen, and discuss the monitoring and follow-up process.

The film is intended for professionals.

Surgery

You and Your New Hip
Available from: Columbia Hospital, Midwest Arthritis Treatment Center, 2025 East Newport Avenue, Milwaukee, Wisconsin 53211. (414) 961-3594.
$60.00 (80 slides and 14-minute audiocassette or 14¾-minute, videotape)
$10.00 booklet

This program offers basic information about the surgical procedure and, in particular, about the rehabilitation process.

INDEX

ABLEDATA, 96

Accent, 86-87

Accent on Living (magazine), 87

Accent on Living Buyer's Guide, 142

Acetaminophen, 47-50

Aceta with Codeine, 47-50, 52

Acetylsalicylic acid (ASA): *See* Aspirin

Acquired immune deficiency syndrome (AIDS), 1

Acromegaly, 22

"Activity and Exercise" (slides and audiocassette), 151-152

Adenoma, 23

Advice for the Patient, 145

"Aging Process, An: Osteoporosis" (film), 149

Aids and Adaptations, 124, 142

Alcohol abuse, risks of, 17, 18

All-American Guide to Calcium-rich Foods, The, 143

Aluminum antacids, 18, 19, 25

Amahen with Codeine, 47-50, 52

Ambulation aids, 127-130

American Academy of Orthopaedic Surgeons, 87, 135-136, 148

American Association of Retired Persons (AARP), 88

American Dietetic Association, 82, 88

American Juvenile Arthritis Organization, 91

American Medical Association, 72, 88-89

American Occupational Therapy Association, 85, 89, 147-148

American Pharmaceutical Association, 89

American Physical Therapy Association, 89-90

American Society for Bone and Mineral Research, 58

Anacin-3 with Codeine, 47-50, 52

Androgens, 47-50, 57

Androsterone, 46, 47-50, 57

Anexia with Codeine, 47-50, 52

Aprons, 123-124

Arteriosclerosis, 23

Arthritis Foundation, 81, 90-91, 143-144

Arthritis Health Professions Association, 90

Arthritis Today (magazine), 90

Arthroplasty, total hip, 67

A.S.A. with Codeine Compound, 47-50, 52

Ascriptin with Codeine, 47-50, 52

Aspirin, 47-52

Auto products, rear view mirror, 131; seat cushion, 130

Balanced diet guidelines, 99-100

Bancap with Codeine, 47-50, 52

Bathing products, 118-120

Bayer, 47-52

Beds and bedding, 122-123

Belchier, John, 138

Biopsy, 45-46

Blood tests, 39-41

Bone, biopsy of, 45-46; components of, 5-8; fractures of: *See* Spinal fractures, Colles fracture, Hip fracture; loss of (osteopenia), 2, 11-13; peak mass of, 37-38; protection of, 71-73; scans of, 43-45

Bone meal, 65

Braces: *See* Orthotics

"Brittle Bones" (film), 149

"Brittle With Age: The Unnecessary Tragedy of Osteoporosis" (videotape), 149-150

Buff-a Comp, 47-50, 52

THE COMPLETE GUIDE TO A LIFETIME OF WELL-BEING BY AMERICA'S MOST TRUSTED HEALTH WRITER

JANE BRODY'S
The New York Times
— GUIDE TO —
PERSONAL HEALTH

Illustrated with graphs and charts, fully indexed and conveniently arranged under fifteen sections:

NUTRITION
EMOTIONAL HEALTH
ABUSED SUBSTANCES
EYES, EARS, NOSE AND
  THROAT
SAFETY
PESKY HEALTH PROBLEMS
COMMON KILLERS
EXERCISE

SEXUALITY AND
  REPRODUCTION
DENTAL HEALTH
ENVIRONMENTAL HEALTH
  EFFECTS
SYMPTOMS
COMMON SERIOUS
  ILLNESSES
MEDICAL CARE

COPING WITH HEALTH PROBLEMS

"Jane Brody's encyclopedia of wellness covers everything."
Washington Post

64121-6/$12.95 US/$16.95 Can